the **food intolerance bible**

DATE DUE

A nut_____ plan to beat food cravings • fatigue

• moo_____ ____ __ disease • headaches • IBS

and deal with food allergies

with over _0 recipes

Antony J. Haynes   Antoinette Savill

Conari Press

First U.S. edition published in 2008 by Conari Press
an imprint of Red Wheel/Weiser, LLC
With offices at:
500 Third Street, Suite 230
San Francisco, CA 94107
www.redwheelweiser.com

10 9 8 7 6 5 4 3 2

First published by Harper*Thorsons* 2005

Library of Congress Cataloging-in-Publication
Data available upon request

ISBN 978-1-57324-359-9

Contents

Introduction

Why Should I Read this Book?

- Do you frequently experience abdominal bloating, even when you haven't over-eaten?
- Do you have symptoms of Irritable Bowel Syndrome?
- Do you have periods during the day when your brain simply does not work as it should?
- Do you suffer from mood swings?
- Are you abnormally tired?

If your answer is 'yes' to one, two or more of these questions, then you may well be experiencing the effects of an intolerance to one or more foods.

You may have picked this book up because you know or suspect that you react adversely to a food or foods. This book is all about food intolerances and how to deal with them and with connected conditions ranging from Chronic Fatigue Syndrome (ME), an overgrowth of the yeast *Candida albicans* (thrush), leaky gut syndrome, excessive stress, parasitic infections, Irritable Bowel Syndrome (IBS), brain fog and even skin conditions such as eczema and respiratory problems such as asthma.

Main Aims of this Book

1. To help you to understand what an intolerance is and discover whether or not you have one (or more) or not

2. You will learn about various ways of confirming your hunch that you have a food intolerance.

3. You will be shown *why* you might have food intolerances, and their causes and connections with other conditions. This will help you identify which of these may be relevant to you in addition to food intolerances. The longer you have had food intolerances, the more likely it is that you will have other, related conditions as well.

4. You will be presented with an action plan for dealing with food intolerance and improving digestion. Putting the action plan to work is made all the more possible by the great recipes prepared by Antoinette, which are free of the most common foods to which people have an intolerance. The recipes are designed to give you a head start and make it as easy as possible to implement the necessary changes in your diet. While this can often require no small effort, if food intolerance is to blame it is vital to helping you overcome your symptoms.

5. To help you improve your health by helping you identify what your food intolerances are, the connected conditions and how to deal with them.

Throughout this book there are questionnaires to help you assess your health and to chart your progress back to better health.

Food Intolerance or Food Allergy?

Before going any further I am going to clarify the distinction between a food allergy and a food intolerance. This has been a source of confusion, not least for those in the health profession.

Originally, the word *allergy* was designated to mean any adverse reaction to any substance inhaled or eaten or coming into contact with the skin, with no specific limitations on the specific nature of the immune reactivity. However, over time, the term *food allergy* has been taken on by allergists and relates to immune reactions mediated by the immunoglobulin E (IgE), which could be to a food or something inhaled or to which we might come into direct physical contact.

Immunoglobulin is a protein that carries out various roles in the body's immune response. There are five: immunoglobulin G, A, M, D and E. Immunoglobulin G (IgG) plays the most significant role of the five in terms of food intolerance, whereas immunoglobulin E (IgE) triggers the most significant reactions. However, not all food intolerance reactions are related to our immune system. For example, tyramine – found in strawberries, cured meats and cheese – can trigger migraines in some people, and this is a brain reaction, not an immune-based one.

Reactions mediated by IgE are referred to as 'true food allergies' – somewhat of a misnomer since it implies that any other type, such as a food intolerance, is 'untrue'. Having said this, these true food allergy reactions are almost always immediate in their manifestation and therefore most often can be traced back to a particular cause. They can often affect health in a significant and rapid manner – swollen lips and tongue, asthma attack – reactions can be life-threatening, which is why great care needs to be taken to avoid the trigger foods or substances. Peanut allergy and shellfish allergy, for example, are perhaps the most well known. Another example is an allergy to latex (rubber) – of allergies triggered just by coming into contact with a substance, this is the one on the most rapid increase. So much of a problem is this specific allergy that at least one hospital has had to change the material of its surgical gloves lest a nurse or doctor succumb to anaphylaxis.

Anaphylaxis is an extreme physical reaction – the reason for which is not fully understood – that often requires adrenaline to counter the extreme stress-reaction caused in the body.

Allergy Is on the Increase

While allergies affect a far smaller proportion of the population than food intolerances, their effects are not insignificant. Unfortunately, allergies are on the increase – some 50 million Americans suffer from some type of allergy on a yearly basis. According to the American Academy of Allergy, Asthma and Immunology, allergy is ranked as the sixth leading cause of chronic disease today, at a cost of $18 billion a year. It is believed that evidence from other Western countries is very similar to that in the US. Two recent estimates of the prevalence of allergy in the US were 9 percent and 16 percent, and the prevalence of the two most common allergies, atopic dermatitis (dry skin, similar to eczema) and allergic rhinitis (persistent runny nose), have been increasing since the mid- to late 1980s.

Food Intolerance Is Escalating, Too

As mentioned, food intolerance is the name for reactions mediated by immunoglobulin G (IgG). These reactions can manifest up to 72 hours after exposure, making the trigger food or substance much more difficult to identify. However, it is worth noting that some food intolerance reactions are not typically mediated by immune reactivity.

While people who suffer from IgG reactions rarely need immediate medical attention, the symptoms can certainly reduce their quality of life and cause long-term illness. The proportion of the population who suffer from at least one food intolerance is as much as 45 percent (and that may be a conservative estimate), making it a significant issue in the nation's health.

Evidence shows that the prevalence of food intolerance is escalating, but because the methodology used to analyze food intolerance is more recent than that for IgE allergy, there are no hard-and-fast figures to compare with the prevalence of decades ago.

> At least 45 percent of the population suffer from food intolerance.

A Wide Range of Symptoms

The range of food intolerance symptoms is as long as it is diverse. You would hardly believe that so many symptoms could be attributable to food intolerance. Simply having interviewed thousands of clients who have avoided certain foods for periods of time and then reintroduced them into their diets, and having listened to their observations about their symptoms, confirms the existence of food intolerance. There is also much evidence today based on the evidence of immunological testing that food intolerance does exist (although, as stated above, not all food intolerances are mediated by immune IgG activity). In spite of all the evidence, however, there are some who refuse to acknowledge food intolerance as an issue, and in particular as a reaction that can cause mental symptoms. This is an issue that I would like to clear up right now, so the rest of this Introduction is devoted to showing you evidence, some of it many years old and some of it very recent, that proves the existence and relevance of food intolerance to a wide range of symptoms.

The Author's Personal Experience

I have suffered with food intolerances myself. I have had a gluten intolerance for years, as measured on more than one occasion with lab tests. To this day I am unable to eat wheat without experiencing unpleasant symptoms. I also have a soy intolerance, this one tested by IgG analysis, that causes sinusitis which only resolves when soy is avoided and which re-emerges when soy is eaten again. I could have figured out what the foods were by observation if I had known what to look for! In hindsight, the reason for these adverse reactions is obvious since I committed the first sin in terms of food intolerance: eating a lot of a certain food on a regular and repetitive basis. You will discover the reasons behind your own intolerances later in this book.

An Ancient Condition

That food can cause adverse symptoms has been appreciated for thousands of years. Herodotus in 460 BC was reported to have said that 'One man's meat is another man's poison.' Hippocrates also identified that stomach upset and skin hives could be caused by drinking milk. It is also something that has been acknowledged and appreciated in medical and academic papers for over a hundred years, but this peer-reviewed literature has not always been given the credence it deserves. It is because of this lack of appreciation for what might be causing a variety of symptoms that uncertainty has been created, and an assumption that such-and-such a symptom must be due to something else, like stress. However, we are now in an age where food intolerance affects at least 45 percent of the population and it has become such an issue that people are seeking out the answers for themselves. Since a food intolerance does not represent a pathology for which there is a medical treatment – by contrast, a food allergy has the potential to do much harm and does require medical attention – there has been much less medical attention focused on this subject. With the march of the masses who suffer from adverse reactions, however, the development of tests, research and investigations into the topic now provide previously unheralded recognition that food intolerance is very real and, unfortunately, a significant factor in many people's health.

I predict, unwillingly and hoping that I will be proved wrong, that with modern lifestyles and our food supply being what they are, food intolerance will increase in the coming years, making it a major cause of unpleasant symptoms for decades to come.

Putting Food Intolerance into Context

However, to place the blame entirely on food intolerance does not properly put the increasing prevalence into context. This assumes that the food is the problem, just like the bacteria is the problem for which the solution is antibiotics. In this example, the germ-warfare approach misses the point which Louis Pasteur, founder of modern-day antibiotics, regretted in his latter days when he said, 'C'est le terrain, pas le germ' which, translated means: It is the host (i.e., the environment or the body) and not the germ (bug, microbe, bacterium, virus) that is important.

In this way, those who believe that stress causes the symptoms have a point, because this can create imbalances within the 'host terrain' (i.e. your body) that permit or make it react inappropriately to foods.

In later chapters you will learn about the connections between stress and food intolerance as well as other underlying issues. These also include imbalances within the digestive system in terms of maldigestion and the graphically-termed 'leaky gut syndrome', and imbalances in the micro-organisms living within our intestines, from yeasts to bacteria and parasites. You will be shown how to address your food intolerances as well as how to address the underlying imbalances. However, it is worth noting that this is not a book designed to assess allergies that require medical attention. More on this in Chapter 1.

Proof of Food Intolerance

There have been observations that food can elicit adverse reactions since the days of Hippocrates. As you will find out in Chapter 1, there are potentially a vast range of symptoms that can be caused by food intolerance reactions. These can be divided into two broad categories: physical (especially digestive) and mental/emotional/behavioral. Since the nature of the symptoms is so diverse, there could potentially be other contributory factors, too, and it is this lack of specificity which has cast some doubt about the phenomenon of food intolerance.

So, can you prove that food intolerance is really the cause of your symptoms? In many cases, you may not need any more proof other than the fact that when you avoid a food you do not get a symptom, but when you eat it you do. In other cases you may have a suspicion about a certain food and therefore an approach which involves elimination/reintroduction – removing the suspected food from your diet and later on reintroducing it into your diet – may serve a useful purpose. (This is *not* a good thing to do if you have a true food allergy, however.) Alternatively, you may wish to implement the pulse-testing method, which will be described later.

However, there are some people who have a potential for multiple food intolerances, which makes an elimination diet and reintroduction difficult to implement. In these cases, a test to tell you which foods you react to would be very useful.

Most people in this situation want to have a firm diagnosis of what is causing, or contributing to, their problems. Equally, doctors also want to have some certainty about what is wrong with their patients so they can make the most apt recommendations. To this end, a degree of proof is always useful – and in Chapter 2 you will find descriptions of a number of accurate tests to help you gather this proof. However, simply testing for immune reactions does not prove in itself that this is the cause of your symptoms; there can be a number of foods to which you are intolerant that cause you no symptoms at all. This is where the avoidance of these foods and a monitoring of symptoms can 'prove' the point nicely. The reintroduction of the offending foods should trigger, in a way that can be easily reproduced, your symptoms.

There have not been many large studies conducted to 'prove' how food intolerance affects various aspects of health. However, there have been studies that show very strong evidence of cause and effect between food intolerance and Irritable Bowel Syndrome (IBS). Indeed, one complaint a medical doctor friend of mine raised about this issue was that he wasn't particularly aware of any 'decent' studies showing that food intolerances really were to blame for a number of symptoms they are claimed to cause. One of the very good reasons for this is that typical medical studies (randomized, placebo-controlled, double-blind studies) are designed to test a drug against a sign or symptom. They are not designed to evaluate the effects of a number of different agents (i.e. foods) on multiple variables (i.e. symptoms). Furthermore, in the case of food intolerance, since the technology for testing is relatively new and because there is no one single test that will accurately identify every single food to which an individual may react, there is difficulty in verifying exactly what foods should be assessed.

Food Intolerance and IBS

IBS was the subject of a recently published study in the respected journal *Gut*, which showed that food intolerances are very much involved in Irritable Bowel Syndrome (IBS). It proved what most complementary therapists have known all their professional lives.

The study involved 150 out-patients with IBS who then had an IgG food intolerance test. They were not shown their results. Seventy-five of the participants were provided with diets that excluded the foods to which they had raised IgG antibodies, while the other 75 participants were given 'sham' diets that excluded foods to which they did *not* have raised IgG levels. A number of symptoms of IBS were compared before and after the diet for 12 weeks. The conclusion was that a diet that eliminates foods to which you have a raised IgG level is indeed effective in reducing the symptoms of IBS.

You may say that this is an obvious finding and you might have expected as much, but the current treatment of IBS is based largely on the use of antispasmodics, antidepressants and medications that alter bowel habit, depending on whether constipation or diarrhea is the predominant problem. This is usually unsatisfactory, however, and encourages patients to seek out alternative treatment. Of course, if food intolerance is to blame for the symptoms, even if not wholly, then the most sensible first-line approach would be to change your diet. This would make recourse to medications the alternative path.

This study represents an important landmark in acknowledging the importance of food in triggering or causing IBS. The patients had experienced symptoms for over a decade and were found to be sensitive to approximately six to seven foods each, on average. Those who fully adhered to the diet showed the greatest improvement.

The reintroduction of the culprit foods also caused their symptoms to get worse. The patients did not embark on anything other than eliminating the culprit foods: They did not take any digestive enzymes, nor anything to restore low stomach-acid levels. They did not supplement with 'friendly' bacteria to combat any possible yeast overgrowth. They did not take active steps to heal their intestinal lining, nor did they take active steps to reduce their stress levels. If these things had been addressed, it is likely that their improvements would have been even greater.

Food Intolerances and Emotional/Behavioral Issues

While it is much more straightforward to understand a link between what you put in your mouth and what happens to your digestion, it is less obvious to see the relationship between what you eat and how you feel in your head, or how you behave. However, as you will see later in this book, there are many food-intolerance symptoms that do not affect digestion.

Your digestive system is designed to absorb tiny components from food to nourish your body. However, it is not always 100 percent successful at preventing the absorption of some matter that can be harmful to or upset the functioning of various organs elsewhere in the body (including the brain). This has long been the subject of published studies, and the basis for clinical treatment. As long ago as 1916, a Dr. Hoobler reported that infants can be intolerant to proteins. Since that time, other studies have identified that reactions to foods can cause hyperactivity, nervousness, learning problems, minimal brain dysfunction, depression, hostility, aggression, periods of confusion and irritability. In those days the distinction between allergy and intolerance had yet to be made, so researchers simply used the word 'allergy' to cover all symptoms and consequences.

If you ever doubted that your irritability, mood swings, clumsiness or brain fog could be the direct result of a food intolerance, then you will swiftly strengthen your resolve when you hear the following accounts.

Case History

The first case to share with you is that of one of my clients, who came to see me with a whole list of complaints. Sally Ann had energy problems, mood problems, digestive problems, skin problems and more. As part of our consultation she completed some questionnaires. One of these, called the Metabolic Screening Questionnaire, is scored on a severity and frequency basis so that the more severe and frequent the symptoms, the higher the score. The maximum score for the 70 symptoms on the questionnaire is 280 – but anything over 80 is indicative of someone with fairly compromised health. A healthy individual may score as little as 10 or less. Sally Ann scored 97. Her doctor was considering antidepressants and hormonal intervention to help her mood, irregular menstrual cycle and painful periods. A thorough examination of her health history and diet and lifestyle revealed that there were many potential areas that could have been contributing to Sally's overall poor state of health. Her diet was particularly high in wheat, which was being consumed at each meal. This was partly due to a lack of time to choose anything different, but none the less Sally was fulfilling the number-one criteria for food intolerance: a high dose and repetitive intake of the same food. When questioned, it was not clear-cut that her increased wheat intake had coincided with her multiple symptoms. However, since the priority was to improve digestive function, I recommended a wheat-free diet.

Sally came back about five weeks later. Her Metabolic Screening Questionnaire was now showing a score of 3 – yes, 3. She looked like a different person: she had lost 8 lb without reducing her caloric intake (in fact, if anything she had eaten more food than usual), her skin had improved, her menstrual cycle had caused her no problems at all and her sex drive had returned. Her poor mood and 'foggy' head had gone, the need to clear her throat had gone, her sore muscles were no longer troubling her, her energy was markedly better and she had no headaches any more. Although in the first few days she had felt markedly worse, this is a well-known sign of withdrawal from a biochemical addiction, and confirmed that she was on the right track.

This was a truly staggering result, and not something I could have predicted. The good news was that no other system in her body had reached a state of exhaustion so that it took only the avoidance of the culprit food to help Sally return to a good state of health. It was also fortunate that she evidently only had one major culprit food. To think that she could have been put on antidepressants, which would not have solved the problem, of course. I wonder how many others with cognitive and mood disorders would benefit from looking at their diets as a source of their symptoms. It is well known, for example, that a large percentage of people who suffer from celiac disease also suffer from bipolar disorder (schizophrenia).

Brain Allergy

Food intolerances can certainly affect the brain. Dr. William Philpott, a psychiatrist and an author of a noteworthy book entitled *Brain Allergies*, has reported that intolerant reactions to foods and pollutants often trigger violent behavior. One of his 12-year-old patients became so aggressive after eating a banana that he picked up a stick and tried to hit another patient.

Temper Tantrums

Nearly 40 years ago, Professor of Psychology Dr. Moyer wrote how a 5-year-old boy with poor speech development had an abnormal EEG (brain scan showing abnormal brainwave patterns) and a temper that was out of control. The boy was found to be intolerant to chocolate, milk and cola, which were then eliminated from his diet for over seven months. The EEG was repeated and found to be normal, and his behavior was much improved. When the culprit foods were then reintroduced, his EEG was once again abnormal and his behavior worsened.

Study into Nervous System Complaints

Two doctors, King and Mandell, conducted a double-blind study of 30 patients in 1978 to test 12 allergens (allergy-inducing triggers) and 6 placebos. The patients reported significantly more nervous system complaints when they were exposed to the allergens compared with the placebos. These included depression, an inability to concentrate, anger, irritability and headaches. Other double-blind studies have confirmed the definite effects of foods on behavior.

Diet, Crime and Delinquency

Alexander Schauss was the Director of the American Institute for Biosocial Research when he wrote his book *Diet, Crime and Delinquency* in 1980. This slim, 108-page volume presents startling evidence that what we eat can have a significant impact on our potential to commit crimes and misbehave. The book is not just about food intolerance, however, but also refers to sugar, toxic metals such as lead, food additives, nutrient insufficiencies, lack of exercise and lack of proper exposure to light.

Summary

Food intolerance has been documented for thousands of years, although it is increasing day by day and is much more prevalent today than ever before. Food intolerance has been well proven to contribute to and even cause the symptoms of

IBS, but it can also cause a wide range of other symptoms, especially those that relate to brain function.

This book is designed to help you to identify whether you have an intolerance, and what this might be doing to you, why you might have intolerances in the first place, and what action you can take to address the situation in order to improve your health.

Part One

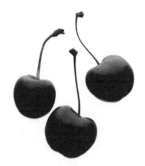

Do I Have a Food Intolerance?

1

How Can I Tell If I Have
a Food Intolerance?

This chapter will help you identify the likelihood of your having a food intolerance. First you will be introduced to 'the usual suspects' – a list of the most common offenders when it comes to food intolerance reactions. Then there is a question-naire to fill in, with a guide for interpreting your score. Then there are details to help you to understand the variety of ways in which food intolerances actually contribute to your symptoms.

First things first. Do you have a food intolerance? Finding out for definite can take a little detective work on your part. This almost always starts with observing any symptoms, which will usually reveal themselves soon after a meal – although given the fact that food intolerance reactions can sometimes be delayed by several hours, it can take a little while before it is possible to identify which foods are causing your symptoms.

The Usual Suspects

This is the name which we have given to the foods and ingredients to which people are most likely to react. These are the foods that have been omitted from the recipes in this book, and the foods against which you should compare your own diet in order to establish whether you consume a high amount of any of them. We've rounded them all up and put them on a list – all the big offenders, all the culprits, taking into account some families such as citrus, nightshade, additives, preservatives and artificial colors. The recipes in this book do not include any of these items, and it has taken Antoinette over a year to get them just right.

1. apples
2. eggplant (nightshade)
3. barley (gluten grain)
4. Brazil nuts
5. broccoli
6. cashews
7. cauliflower
8. chilies (nightshade)
9. chocolate
10. citrus fruits (such as oranges, limes, lemons, grapefruit)
11. cola nuts
12. corn
13. cow's-milk products (milk, cheese, yogurt, butter)
14. cucumbers
15. durum wheat
16. eggs
17. broad beans
18. honey
19. kidney beans
20. lentils
21. malt
22. MSG (mono-sodium glutamate)
23. oats (gluten grain)
24. peas
25. peanuts
26. pork
27. potatoes (nightshade)
28. rye (gluten grain)
29. sheep's cheese and milk
30. soy
31. sweet green peppers (nightshade)
32. sweet red peppers (nightshade)
33. sugar
34. tomatoes (nightshade)

35. vinegar
36. wheat (gluten grain)
37. yeast
38. tea
39. coffee
40. all gluten grains

41. all members of the nightshade
    family
42. all food additives
43. all food preservatives
44. all artificial colors
45. tobacco

> With the exception of gluten and sugar, preservatives, additives and artificial colors, if it turns out you were not intolerant to any of these, you can of course still eat them. While you are finding out which if any of these culprits apply to you, you can continue to enjoy Antoinette's recipes, which contain none of these ingredients.

While this is the most comprehensive attempt yet to prepare recipes that omit foods that might trigger an adverse reaction, the recipes are still not going to be suitable for everyone, so please be warned. We have not avoided all nuts and seeds, for example. In addition, there are bound to be individual items not in this list that a test may identify as a problem for you. If this turns out to be the case, we hope that it will be possible for you to identify the recipes that include this culprit and choose different meals, or be able to replace that individual ingredient.

To help alert you to the most likely culprits within this list, here are the Top Five Usual Suspects to consider as a trigger for your symptoms:

1. cow's-milk products
2. gluten grains (wheat, oats, rye, barley)

3. soy

4. sugar

5. yeast

For children the list is slightly different:

1. cow's-milk products

2. food additives and colorings

3. gluten grains (wheat, oats, rye, barley)

4. sugar

5. yeast

This 'Usual Suspects list' will be referred to throughout this book.

Now, your next task is to find out if you are suffering from food intolerance.

The Food Intolerance Questionnaire

If you regularly have any of the 80-plus symptoms on the following questionnaire, this could be a sign that you have a food intolerance, particularly if you know of no other reason why your symptoms might be present. Since you have already chosen to read this book you may already be wise to this possibility. Perhaps this list could also help a family member or friend who you know suffers from symptoms but does not know the cause.

Please complete the questionnaire below and see what the score reveals. The questionnaire can also be printed out directly from the website:

www.thefoodintolerancebible.com

Be sure to see your doctor if you have any persistent health problem so that it can be investigated medically. Just because you have one or more of the symptoms below does *not* mean that they must be caused by an adverse reaction to certain foods.

If you answer 'yes' to any of the following, score one or two points depending on the specific question (some symptoms are more relevant to food intolerances, so they score 2 points), as shown below.

SECTION ONE – DIGESTIVE SYMPTOMS

Do you suffer on a regular basis (i.e. more than 3 times a week) from any of the following?

- abdominal bloating/distension (2)
- abdominal cramps (2)
- abdominal or stomach pain (2)
- burping after eating certain foods
- catarrh (mucus) (2)
- difficulty gaining weight
- difficulty losing weight
- enuresis (bed-wetting) (2)
- excess wind (flatulence)
- gallbladder problems (difficulty digesting fats)
- Gastro-oesophageal Reflux Disease (GORD) (2)
- glue ear (otitis media) (2)
- gritty feeling in the eyes (2)
- hemorrhoids (piles) (2)
- indigestion (recurring) (2)

- inexplicable weight gain or weight loss
- irregular bowel motions (e.g. constipation or diarrhoea) (2)
- Irritable Bowel Syndrome (IBS) (2)
- itchy anus
- itchy, red ears (2)
- metallic taste in the mouth (2)
- mouth ulcers (2)
- nausea
- persistent need to clear your throat/sore throat (2)
- post-nasal drip (2)
- rhinitis (runny nose) (2)
- sinusitis (2)
- sneezing – frequent (2)
- water retention (edema)

(20 x 2 = 40)

(9 x 1 = 9)

Sub-total/maximum =   /49

SECTION TWO – MENTAL, EMOTIONAL AND NERVOUS SYSTEM SYMPTOMS

- addictions
- aggressive outbursts
- anxiety
- Attention Deficit Disorder/ADHD (2)
- behavioral problems (2)
- blankness or momentary difficulty finding the right word(s) (2)

- blurred vision (2)
- brain fog (2)
- changes in handwriting (2)
- clumsiness (2)
- confusion
- constant hunger (2)
- dark circles under your eyes (2)
- depression
- dilated blood vessels in your cheeks and nose (2)
- dizziness
- dyslexia (2)
- fidgeting
- foggy head (2)
- food cravings (2)
- headaches
- hyperactivity (especially in children) (2)
- inability to think clearly (2)
- insomnia
- irritability
- lack of motivation/get up and go
- migraines (2)
- mood swings
- palpitations
- panic attacks
- phobias
- poor concentration
- racing pulse
- restless legs syndrome

- slurred speech
- spaciness (2)
- tenseness
- tinnitus (ringing in the ears) (2)
- uncharacteristic inability to make decisions

(18 x 2 = 36)

(21 x 1 = 21)

Sub-total/maximum =   /57

SECTION THREE – OVERT PHYSICAL SIGNS AND SYMPTOMS

- abnormal physical weakness or tiredness
- aching muscles and joints for no good reason (2)
- arthritis
- asthma
- chronic infections
- eczema
- fibromyalgia (diagnosed by a physical therapist or doctor) (2)
- hives (urticaria) (2)
- itching (2)
- painful joints in which the pain moves from one joint to another (2)
- painful joints not associated with excessive use (2)
- pimples or acne (that are not hormonally related)
- psoriasis (2)
- rheumatoid arthritis

- rough, dry skin
- skin rashes (for no other known reason) (2)
- wheezing

(8 x 2 = 16)

(9 x 1 = 9)

Sub-total/maximum =   /25

WHAT IS YOUR SCORE?

Section One	*/49*
Section Two	*/57*
Section Three	*/25*
Overall Total	*/131*

INTERPRETING YOUR SCORE

Essentially, the higher your score, the more likely it is that your reactions are the result of a food intolerance. (The individual section scores are important in themselves, since, for example, they may highlight digestive problems that are distinct from food intolerances – more about this later.)

Note: Do not reintroduce a food if you suffer with a severe physical reaction such as wheezing or asthma, without medical supervision.

If Your Score Is Between 0 and 15

This is a low score and not particularly indicative of food intolerance. Please check your diet to see if it contains many of the 'Usual Suspects' and avoid *two* of the most frequently-eaten foods, replacing them with alternatives. Avoid these foods for two weeks and observe whether your symptoms improve. If your symptoms have improved, then avoid these foods for a further two weeks (one month in total). Then reintroduce the foods, one at a time, allowing four days in between. Eat a normal portion of the food. Observe whether any of your symptoms return. Sometimes foods continue to trigger reactions even after you have avoided them for a period of time, sometimes not. However, even if there is no worsening of symptoms, it is suggested that you do not eat the culprit food(s) every day, in case you re-create the original intolerance symptoms. If a food triggers symptoms again, then avoid the food completely for two months and repeat the reintroduction process. If the symptoms persist after this time, continue to avoid the food, but investigate other conditions detailed in later chapters of this book. This will be helped by completing the relevant questionnaires.

If, after the two weeks, your symptoms have not improved by avoiding the two main potential culprits, then reintroduce them in the manner described. Sometimes this can still trigger other symptoms – or worsen the ones you already have – which highlights that the specific food is a culprit food and needs to be avoided for a month. However, because your overall symptoms have not improved, this indicates that other intolerances, or even other conditions, may exist. If this is the case, you are recommended to *follow the next paragraph's instructions AND complete the questionnaires in the chapters that follow*, to help identify any other conditions you may be suffering from.

Since your score is so low, there is no strong indication for you to undertake a food-intolerance test at this stage.

If Your Score Is Between 16 and 25

This is a moderate score and reflects that you have too many symptoms to be in optimal health. You need to do something different in order to improve your symptoms, and a food intolerance investigation should be carried out as part of this process. Please check your diet to see if it contains many of the 'Usual Suspects' and avoid the top *four* of these (in terms of regularity and volume of consumption – e.g. wheat, dairy, sugar and tomatoes – or whatever you identify in your diet), for two weeks.

Also, start the Digestive Support Plan, as detailed in Part 3.

If your symptoms have improved, then avoid them for a further two weeks (one month in total). Then reintroduce the foods, one at a time, allowing four days in between. Eat a normal portion of the food. Observe whether any of your symptoms return. Sometimes foods continue to trigger reactions after you have avoided them for a period of time, sometimes not. However, even if there is no worsening of symptoms, it is suggested that you do not eat the culprit food(s) every day in case you re-create the original intolerance symptoms. If a food triggers symptoms again, then avoid that food completely for two months before repeating the reintroduction process. If the symptoms persist after this time, continue to avoid the food, but investigate other conditions detailed in Part 2. This will be helped by completing the relevant questionnaires.

If, after the two weeks, your symptoms have not improved by avoiding the *four* main potential culprits, then reintroduce them in the manner described. Sometimes this can still trigger symptoms – or worsen the ones you already have. This highlights that the specific food is a culprit food and needs to be avoided for a month. However, because your overall symptoms have not improved, this indicates that other intolerances – or even other conditions – may exist. If this is the case, you are recommended to *follow the next paragraph's instructions AND complete the questionnaires later in this book to help you identify the other conditions that may be contributing to your symptoms.*

If you do not score highly in the other questionnaires (high scores are indicated at the end of the questionnaires and in Part 3), then you should undertake *either* The Pulse Test, which is detailed in Appendix I, *or* a food intolerance test, discussed in Chapter 2 and detailed in Appendix II.

If you *do* score highly on any of the other questionnaires, then you are recommended to follow the Action Plan detailed in Part 3.

If Your Score Is Between 26 and 35

This is a score that suggests problems relating to food intolerance quite strongly. You should follow the instructions below and consider proceeding with the actions detailed in Option 2 or Option 3.

Start the Digestive Support Plan. Please check your diet to see if it contains many of the 'Usual Suspects' and avoid the top *six* of these (e.g. cow's-milk products, gluten grains, soy, sugar, yeast – or whatever you identify in your diet) and replace with alternatives, using the recipes in this book to help you. Do this for one month, then repeat the questionnaire to monitor your progress. If there is no progress, review Part 2 and complete the questionnaires there, if you have not already, to help identify any other conditions you may have that are connected to food intolerance. Continue with the Digestive Support Plan, and consider proceeding with Option 2 or Option 3 below.

Option 2

To obtain more certainty about the true state of your food intolerances, undertake The Pulse Test as discussed in Chapter 2 and detailed in Appendix I. This does not cost anything, but requires some time and attention.

Option 3

Have one of the two types of food intolerance blood tests, as described in Chapter 2 and detailed in Appendix II, whichever is most convenient for you. This costs money but requires little time.

I Know My Test Results – What Should I Do Now?

If you have done a lab test and you now have a list of culprit foods, then eliminate them for three whole months – the recipes in this book will help you with what you can eat instead. Once a month during this time, review your symptom scores by redoing the questionnaire (which is also available on-line). For most people, the symptoms should diminish over a matter of weeks, and therefore you should see improved scores each time you retake the questionnaire.

After three months, plan a reintroduction schedule, reintroducing individual foods, four days apart, and consuming a normal, moderate portion of the food and observing your symptoms. If you still react to a food, then avoid it for a further three months. For those foods that you do not react to, eat them every third or fourth day. Continue the Digestive Support Plan for the first three months, after which, if your symptoms have improved, you can stop. If symptoms emerge because you have stopped the Digestive Support Plan, then begin it again for one more month.

If your score in The Food Intolerance Questionnaire does not drop to below 15 when you exclude these foods, then consider that other imbalances may well exist, and review your answers to the questionnaires in Part 2 with the intention of addressing the other most significant conditions present, such as stress or leaky gut syndrome, for example. Since it is not practical to follow more than two plans at any one time, follow the Plan indicated by the results of the questionnaires. Even if you score very highly in all the other questionnaires, then choose the test with the highest ranking, as detailed in Part 3.

If Your Score Is Between 36 and 50

This score is strongly suggestive of problems relating to food intolerance. After you have seen a doctor to rule out other medical conditions, do one type of testing for food intolerances and follow the Digestive Support Plan. The Pulse Test or blood test are discussed in Chapter 2, and detailed in Appendices I and II respectively.

In addition, your score is also strongly indicative of the presence of something other than food intolerances, so complete the questionnaires in Part 2 and undertake the relevant Action Plan as detailed in Part 3.

I Know My Test Results – What Should I Do Now?

Once you have your lab test results, exclude the culprit foods for three whole months – the recipes in this book will help you with what you can eat instead. Once a month during this time, review your symptom scores by retaking the questionnaire (which is also available on-line, see page 21). For most people, symptoms should have diminished over a matter of weeks, and therefore you should see improved scores in your questionnaire each time you retake it.

To determine if you can eat any of the tested positive foods again with impunity, after three months plan a reintroduction schedule. Consume a normal, moderate portion of each food every four days, and observe your symptoms. If you still react to a food, then avoid it for a further three months. Even for those foods you do not react to, don't start eating them again every day – eat them every third or fourth day so that you do not re-create the intolerance.

Continue the Digestive Support Plan for the first three months; if your symptoms have improved after this, then stop. If symptoms emerge because you have stopped the Digestive Support Plan, then start it again for another month. If you feel that the Digestive Support Plan is helping you, there's no reason you can't continue it indefinitely – though you should take a break from it every few months so you can make sure it still meets your needs.

If your score does not drop to below 15 even after you have excluded the culprit foods for three months, then other imbalances may also exist. Retake the questionnaires for other conditions to see if your scores have dropped. If you do not score less than half what you did first-time round, you need to double-check that you are avoiding the culprit foods in all their forms. You should also:

i) Go and see a nutritionist, armed with all this information, or:

ii) Take a test for Intestinal Permeability (see Appendix III) if you have not already done so; if positive, follow the Gut Lining Support Plan
if negative, then:

iii) Take the next most important relevant test as highlighted by the questionnaires (e.g. Adrenal Stress Profile, Stool Analysis or Dysbiosis Profile).
You may still need some help in addressing imbalances, so do seek out a good nutritionist near you (see Resources chapter, pages 333–42).

I Scored Low in Section 1, But High in Sections 2 and 3 of the Questionnaire
If your scores are heavily weighted in favor of the mental symptoms or physical

signs and symptoms rather than the digestive symptoms, then you should take the test that measures Intestinal Permeability (see Appendix III). If positive, then follow the Gut Lining Support Plan (pages 158–9).

If Your Score Is 51 to 70

This score is strongly suggestive of problems relating to food intolerance as well as at least one other significant imbalance. After you have seen a doctor to rule out other medical conditions, follow the Digestive Support Plan and schedule either a Pulse Test or other lab tests – as discussed in Chapter 2 and detailed in Appendices I and II respectively.

In addition, take the next most relevant test for you, based on your scores to the questionnaires in Part 2. If there are two areas that are strongly indicated, then it is advised that you do two tests, not one. For example, without knowing for sure if parasites are present (Comprehensive Parasitology) or whether your cortisol level is very high (Adrenal Stress Profile), it may prove more than difficult to make any headway and improve your health, let alone resolve your food intolerances.

Certainly, a trial away from the foods you consume which best match the top five 'Usual Suspects' would be important, but first you need to make sure what else is having a detrimental effect on your health.

I Scored Low in Section 1, But High in Sections 2 and 3 of the Questionnaire

If your scores are heavily weighted in favor of the mental symptoms or physical signs and symptoms rather than the digestive symptoms, then you should take the urine test to measure your Intestinal Permeability (see pages 109–11). If positive, then follow the Gut Lining Support Plan (pages 158–9).

If Your Score Is Above 71

It is hoped that no one scores this high, but if you do, I'd recommend you do a food intolerance test and seek the help of a qualified nutritionist. Do take along all the information from this book with you, including the completed questionnaires, as this can only help.

Your score is strongly suggestive of problems relating to food intolerance as well as at least one other significant imbalance. Please also make sure that you have seen your doctor to rule out any other underlying medical condition.

Alternatively, if you have already seen your doctor, you could follow the guidelines above for those who score between 51 and 70.

Food Intolerance Questionnaire Score Summary

Your Score		Action
Total	= 0–15	Exclude the top two 'Usual Suspects'
Total	= 16–25	Exclude the top four 'Usual Suspects'; follow the Digestive Support Plan
Total	= 26–35	Exclude top six 'Usual Suspects'; follow the Digestive Support Plan
Total	= 36–50	Food Intolerance Lab Test OR Pulse Test and avoid the identified culprit foods; follow the Digestive Support Plan and the plan that combats any other identified condition
Total	= 51–70	Food Intolerance Lab Test and next most relevant test, and avoid the identified culprit foods; follow the Digestive Support Plan
Total	= >71	Food Intolerance Lab Test and visit a nutritionist

Total   = > 36   but combined score for Sections 2 and 3 is more than double
                      that for Section 1: Intestinal Permeability Test

---

EXPLAINING THE SECTION SCORES

You scores in each of the three different sections do not wholly alter the process of identifying food intolerance, nor which Plan you should follow. However, they do help you distinguish between the different effects food intolerances are having in your body, as well as potentially highlighting other causes of your symptoms. This also simplifies completing the questionnaire next time, since you may only have to repeat the one relevant section rather than the entire questionnaire.

Section One is clearly mostly related to digestive issues, whereas Sections Two and Three refer to things going on elsewhere in the body. If your total score is 36 or more, and your score for Sections Two and Three (added together) is twice that of Section One, then you could have a leaky gut but without the associated digestive symptoms. In this instance it would be worthwhile testing your intestinal permeability (see urine test, Appendix III). However, please note that it is not worth taking this test if other markers within the digestive system are going to be measured and treated first.

If your score in Section One is half or less that of the combined totals of Sections Two and Three, then take the Intestinal Permeability test (Appendix III).

A Question of Severity

The questionnaires do not take severity into account, so if you have a severe symptom or set of symptoms, then even if you have not scored highly in the questionnaire please ask your doctor to investigate the matter.

Similarly, even if you have only some of the above symptoms (particularly those that score 2 points in The Food Intolerance Questionnaire) but their effect is severe, this is also worth further investigation. It may certainly be worthwhile analysing your diet to see how many of the Usual Suspects you eat on a regular basis, or eat a lot of. You may also want to think about taking a pulse test, and also one of the other food intolerance lab tests described in detail later in this book.

On-line Questionnaires

If you'd like a print-out of any of the questionnaires in this book, please visit www.thefoodintolerancebible.com.

How Does Food Intolerance Cause My Symptoms?

This is a major source of confusion and controversy. It is still not completely understood how food intolerance causes symptoms, though that's not to say that the methods of identification are inaccurate. It's just that the range of different reactions to foods makes it impossible to use a single method of testing to categorize food intolerance neatly into one box.

IMMUNE REACTIVITY

Your food intolerance reactions are mostly mediated by your immune system, as a result of the delicate interactions between food, your digestive tract, white blood cells and food-specific antibodies called immunoglobulins, as mentioned in the Introduction. There are five types of immunoglobulin: IgA, IgD, IgE, IgG and IgM. The molecules of food to which the body makes antibodies are referred to as *antigens*. Given that you eat three to four times a day, effectively exposing your body to foreign substances in the process, the food you eat easily represents the single biggest antigenic challenge confronting the human immune system – so perhaps it should not be surprising that your body would make antibodies to foods as often as to any other 'foreign' matter it encounters.

HYPERSENSITIVITY

Hypersensitivity reactions have been categorized in various ways, although even this does not always help us when it comes to determining the most appropriate tests that should be done. Nor does this change that fact that you need to avoid the culprit food(s) and address other aspects of your health as necessary. Categorizing reactions is of much more use to scientists and medical experts involved in the field. However, showing you the different categories will help you understand why symptoms such as yours may have been misunderstood or misdiagnosed in the past. It will also help you understand why some tests can be wholly inappropriate for you and your symptoms.

These are the classifications for hypersensitivity reactions:

Type I - Immediate IgE reactions

Type II - Cytotoxic antibody-mediated reactions

Type III - Delayed-onset, mainly IgG-mediated reactions

Type IV - Cell-mediated and T Cell-mediated reactions which may also involve IgG reactions

Now let's take a look at each one in more detail.

Type I - Immediate IgE reactions

These reactions occur within two hours. Food molecules (antigens) bind to IgE antibodies that have already been made in the body, and trigger the release of molecules such as histamine and leukotrienes. It is these substances that cause symptoms – and in this case they are the classic allergy symptoms, such as swollen lips or tongue. Since this represents a potentially life-threatening situation, and is not the type of allergy that is the focus of this book, you need to see your doctor about this.

IgE Food Allergy Checklist
1. Gasping for air (throat swells up); coughing, wheezing, difficulty breathing
2. Swelling of the lips, face or eyes; flushing
3. Severe nausea, vomiting, diarrhea or severe abdominal cramps/pain
4. Weakness or inability to stand/walk
5. Collapse or near-collapse
6. Sudden drop in blood pressure
7. Loss of consciousness

The result of the IgE-mediated reactions are almost always unpleasant and also include nasal irritation, sinus congestion, hives (urticaria) or eczema, arthritis, intestinal inflammation, headaches or 'spaciness' or loss of memory. Estimates put the prevalence of immediate hypersensitivity reactions to 10–15 percent of all food allergy and intolerance reactions.

Immuno Laboratories offers various tests – see Appendix II.

Type II - Cytotoxic Antibody-mediated Reactions
This is a delayed-response reaction which involves either IgG or, less commonly, IgM. The reactions are known as cytotoxic because the cell to which the antigen is bound is actually destroyed. An example of this type of reaction occurs in hemolytic anemia, in which red cell platelets are destroyed. Another is the type of reaction to penicillin. It is estimated that at least 75 percent of all food allergy reactions are accompanied by cell destruction.

Type III - Delayed-onset, Mainly IgG-mediated Reactions

The prime immune cell involved in these reactions is IgG. The reason for the delay in the reaction is because time is needed for the immune complex to form. The immune complex is made up of an antigen (food molecule) and an antibody, and triggers the release of inflammatory molecules from various tissues in the body, thereby causing inflammation. If these immune complexes are not eliminated from the body they can deposit in tissues and cause injury. The more immune complexes there are, and the more histamine and other 'amines' that are produced by the body, the more likely there will be tissue damage. An estimated 80 percent of food intolerance reactions involve IgG.

Type IV - Cell-mediated and T Cell-mediated Reactions Which May Also Involve IgG Reactions

This type of reaction is also a delayed one, and is usually mediated by T-Cells, a special kind of immune cell. They occur when an antigen comes into contact with your skin, respiratory tract or gastrointestinal tract. Within two to four days of contact, inflammation can produce symptoms. This does not involve any anti-bodies. This type of reaction is involved in tuberculosis, viral infections, contact dermatitis (such as poison ivy) and allergic colitis (inflammation in the colon).

REACTIONS TRIGGERED BY OTHER FACTORS

There are also many reactions to food that are not triggered by your immune system. Instead, the reaction is caused by inflammatory mediators such as histamine, something most people have heard of, and prostaglandins, leukotrienes, serotonin, platelet-activating factor, kinins and more besides.

- Some foods can influence the release of these inflammatory mediators or can even contain high levels of substances that provoke intolerant-like reactions:

sauerkraut, sausage, wine, tuna, spinach and tomatoes all contain a high level of histamine.

- Other foods cause the release of histamine: molluscs, crustaceans, strawberries, tomatoes, chocolate, bananas and papayas (which contain enzymes called proteases) and alcohol.
- Other foods contain amines (protein groups) such as tyramine, which have a vasoactive effect – meaning they affect the constriction of blood vessels: cabbage, cheese, citrus fruit, seafood, strawberries, salami and other cured meats, and potatoes.

Summary

You now know that there are many different symptoms that can indicate the presence of a food intolerance. You will also have gone a long way toward figuring out whether you have food intolerances by completing the questionnaire and checking to see if you eat a lot of the 'Usual Suspects' – and in particular the top-five culprit foods. You have also been given guidelines on what to do on the basis of your score though you may also need to rule out a number of other related conditions that you will find out more about in Part 2. Part 3 will then help you with Action Plans for combating your symptoms and their underlying causes, while the recipe section (Part 4) provides alternatives to your potential culprit foods.

In this chapter you have also learned of the complex and varied mechanisms behind food intolerance and allergy, and why diagnosing the problem can be so difficult. The next chapter is all about the tests available to help with a diagnosis of food intolerance.

2

What Tests Can Confirm
Food Intolerance?

Please note that if the results for any of the tests in this book are positive, you are advised to notify your doctor.

As mentioned in Chapter 1, diagnosing a food intolerance is not an exact science because of the many different types of reactions that can occur. It is possible for an individual to have more than just one type of reaction to a food, and so can be difficult to pin down exactly what is causing symptoms.

This is not to say that the tests available are inaccurate; it is more a question of whether they can pick up everything you are reacting to. No one single test will do this for you, except perhaps the elimination diet followed by reintroduction and a careful observation of your symptoms.

There will always be some for whom a certain test works wonderfully well, while others will find it of no help at all. While this charge can be leveled at any kind of test, this makes it all the more important to learn a little more about a method of testing before trusting it absolutely. Also, with food intolerance testing it is necessary to put the results into context with an individual's particular symptoms and overall health. This is why it is useful to learn about any studies that have been conducted on these tests and what medical experts have to say.

This chapter tells you about the ways you can verify the presence of a food intolerance through some means of testing, which takes various forms including laboratory testing, pulse testing, elimination diets with reintroduction challenges, Vega tests, kinesiology, skin prick test, RAST (Radio Allergo Sorbent Test, now outdated) and electroacupuncture (EAV). This chapter reviews the range of tests and some of the studies that have been conducted to ascertain their efficacy, with the aim of helping you decide which test is most appropriate for you.

What Is ELISA?

ELISA is a technique of analysis used for a variety of tests, not just food intolerance. The letters stand for Enzyme-Linked ImmunoSorbent Assay. It is a highly accurate technique. Many food intolerance tests use this technology, including those recommended in this book (see Resources chapter).

Advantages and Disadvantages of Allergy and Intolerance Tests

TEST	Advantages	Disadvantages
Pulse test	No cost. Sensitive to all kinds of adverse reactions to food. Much research evidence.	Time consuming; results difficult to confirm. Requires thorough compliance. Few clinical studies.
Exclusion/Challenge	No cost. Sensitive to all kinds of adverse reactions to food. Experience of symptoms is very powerful.	Time consuming with little way of confirming results. Requires high compliance. Possible danger of severe reaction.
Skin Prick	Good for inhalant substances. Good for IgE reactions.	Poor sensitivity to food intolerances (which are not IgE reactions).
Vega Test	Sensitive to all kinds of adverse reactions to food.	Few clinical studies. May vary from one doctor to another.
EAV	Possibly sensitive to all kinds of adverse reactions to food.	Unknown scientific basis.

Kinesiology	Sensitive to all kinds of adverse reactions to food. Easily applied. Immediate.	Few clinical studies. Poor evidence in some studies. May vary from one doctor to another.
RAST		Outdated – superseded by ELISA Poor sensitivity to food intolerances
ELISA IgG	Convenient (1 test). Good sensitivity to IgG reactions. Much clinical evidence. Good research evidence of sensitivity in IBS.	Less evidence of use in conditions other than IBS. Expensive. IgG results may vary from lab to lab depending on source of antigens used.
Chemical Mediators from white blood cells (e.g. FACTest)	Convenient (1 test). Sensitive to more than simply IgG reactions. Much clinical evidence. Good evidence of sensitivity in IBS.	Less evidence of use in conditions other than IBS. Expensive.

The trouble is, no test that is useful for diagnosing food intolerances has had masses of solid research performed on it. One of the main reasons for this is that they are not mainstream medical tests for which large-scale studies are conducted, and they are very expensive to undertake. Also, the nature of such studies usually favors the use of one active substance (e.g. drug) on one outcome (e.g.

pain) which does not lend itself well to assessing multiple food intolerances with multiple symptoms.

Now let's take a look in more detail at each of these.

The Pulse Test

This is a wonderfully useful test, and I would recommend it for monitoring your reactions to different foods. If your heart beats faster after having eaten a certain food (complete instructions are given in Appendix I), this indicates that it may be a culprit food for you. When you test your pulse on a regular basis, it gives you great feedback and soon you will have confidence in the method.

This is a method which requires attention to detail, concentration and application, but the results can be very rewarding.

The Elimination Diet

This is the traditional method for identifying foods to which you have an adverse reaction. There are variations on the theme, but the most strict type is to avoid all food and go on a water fast only for three days, and then introduce lamb and pears only. You do this for a period of time, from two to four weeks, then reintroduce individual foods one by one, with a gap of a number of days (usually four) in between each reintroduction. If the avoidance of a food leads to a reduction in symptoms and its reintroduction leads to a worsening of symptoms, then you are intolerant to that food.

This approach requires time and attention – and it is recommended that you record your reactions in writing as you go.

Following this method is difficult, and there are also problems related to malnutrition and care of the individual who embarks on this process. It is also difficult to confirm results with other modes of testing. With multiple food intolerances, it may prove very difficult to identify them all, since your symptoms may not improve even if you do avoid culprit foods because other foods contributing to your symptoms have not been avoided, even in the limited exclusion diet. This is where it may be best to consider a blood test.

Additionally, if there are complicating conditions as highlighted in Part 2, it may not be possible to identify whether symptoms are related to the food or to something else, such as a bacterial overgrowth or a liver detoxification problem. Lastly, this type of testing is not so suitable for unmasking delayed food intolerances as opposed to immediate reactions – which would in any case require medical attention.

A variation on this type of approach has been outlined in Chapter 1, and involves 'simply' eliminating the most obvious culprit foods from the Usual Suspects list for a period of time and then reintroducing them one by one. This is much more straightforward and produces good results without the extreme measures of the full Elimination Diet. The recipes and Resources in this book should greatly help you to implement this simpler approach.

Again, it is important to warn you that those with more serious conditions such as asthma should not undertake this approach because it is possible that reintroducing culprit foods will trigger a more severe reaction than when you were consuming them every day.

Elimination-Challenge Method Proves Useful in IBS
Over 20 years ago, the *Lancet* published a study which showed that food intoler-

ance affects the symptoms of Irritable Bowel Syndrome. Twenty-one patients with IBS followed a strict elimination diet (no other tests were done) which consisted of one meat, one fruit and distilled or spring water for one week. For 14 of the patients, the symptoms disappeared. Then the patients reintroduced single foods, one at a time, and recorded their reactions. The following foods evoked symptoms: wheat (9 patients), corn (5), dairy products (4), coffee (4), tea (3), citrus fruits (2). Biopsies were carried out on the nine cases of wheat intolerance and proved that they did not have celiac disease. Their blood was analyzed, and this confirmed that the symptoms were mediated at least in part by prostaglandins, but that an immunological mechanism did not seem to be involved.

Since complying with such a strict elimination diet may be very difficult for some, it makes it extremely difficult to use this type of testing method for every patient.

Skin Prick
This test is not suitable for food intolerance testing.

Vega Test
I know colleagues who use the Vega test and they have consistently good results with their patients. There is not much scientific evidence in the way of trials – but then this is true for many tests for food intolerance.

Electroacupuncture According to Voll (EAV)
Similar comments apply to this as to Kinesiology and Vega testing, although this is less commonly available than either of the other two.

Kinesiology
Muscle-testing can prove very effective as a means of testing for food intolerance.

Again, I know of practitioners who have a great deal of success with it, but there are also studies which highlight the inconsistencies of this technique.

RAST

This test is not suitable for food intolerance testing.

ELISA IgG

This method has been shown to be effective by a small number of studies that have been carried out. However, you may recall that not all food intolerances are mediated by IgG reactions, and while 80 percent is a high figure you could miss some extremely important reactions to foods that are causing your symptoms by another means. There is much clinical evidence for this type of test, although one question with IgG testing is the source of the antigens, which could be something other than the foods you eat. This explains why one lab's results can vary from another, even from blood drawn from the same person on the same day.

Cellular Mediators (i.e. FACT)

There is at least one study, along with much clinical evidence and medical support, that validate the efficacy of this test. Many find it appealing because it examines the inflammatory cascade which may be triggered by more than just one type of immunoglobulin (i.e. IgG) and which occurs in non-immune mediated reactions.

Food Allergen Cellular Test (FACT)

This is a test (also known as ALCAT) that measures cellular mediators released from white blood cells, such as histamine and leukotrienes (which can be 10,000 more inflammatory than histamine), when they are exposed to food allergens. Contact Immuno Laboratories (see Appendix II) for more information.

It is already known that inflammatory chemicals are responsible for a number of symptoms associated with food intolerance. ELISA technology is used in the testing procedure to measure leukotriene release very precisely. Since leukotrienes are released in the face of a number of different types of intolerance/allergic reaction, including IgE and IgG as well as other non-immune-related responses, the test is therefore thought to be capable of detecting a wide range of reactions.

This test has been the subject of a study involving 200 participants with clearly defined symptoms. On the basis of the results, each participant was given a four-day rotational diet plan which excluded those foods that had appeared positive in the FACT. They followed this diet for three months. Their symptoms had included rheumatism/joint or muscle pain, fatigue, lethargy, mood fluctuation, eczema, itchy skin, acne; migraine, headache, IBS, diarrhea, constipation, bloating, stomach cramps; weight problems, sinus congestion, rhinitis and Chronic Fatigue Syndrome.

At the end of the three months, the participants reported on the status of their symptoms in terms of frequency and severity. The improvements across the board were noteworthy, and are shown below:

Symptom Completed	Number Percentage	Number and Percentage of Participants Who Showed Improvement
Rheumatism/joint or muscle pain	8	7 (88%)
Fatigue, lethargy, mood fluctuation	38	35 (97%)
Eczema, itching skin, acne	16	13 (81%)
Migraine, headache	11	9 (82%)
IBS, diarrhea, constipation, bloating, stomach cramps	80	71 (93%)
Weight problems	26	24 (92%)

Sinus congestion, rhinitis	4	3 (75%)
Chronic Fatigue Syndrome	2	1 (50%)

These improvements are impressive, and highlight the significant association of food intolerance and IBS, something noted in the 1982 *Lancet* study cited earlier. In a clinical setting, the outcome of patients who have excluded the positive foods identified by this test are similar to the impressive figures shown above. An experienced and extremely knowledgeable nutritionist, Xandria Williams, has used this test for years:

> *I have used a range of different food intolerance tests including IgG Elisa and Cytotoxic, but in my clinical experience the best results have been achieved when using the FACTest.*
>
> Xandria Williams,
> nutritional practitioner and best-selling author of *Living with Allergies*

In a more recent analysis of food intolerance testing and IBS, described in the Introduction, similarly encouraging results were found.

It would seem that if you have IBS you would do well to avoid the foods to which you are intolerant, and if you cannot find out which foods these are, then a test measuring either IgG or cellular mediators (e.g. the FACTest) would be advisable. The test in this instance would almost certainly save you time and effort in determining which foods to avoid.

The time factor is one of the most important advantages of having a blood test for food intolerances, certainly compared with elimination diets, which are discussed below.

The Usual Suspects

Before you find out more about lab testing, there are a number of things you can do at home to determine if you have a problem with a food intolerance. First, you can make keen observations about how you feel when you eat a certain food, and at the same time compare your intake against the Usual Suspects list in Chapter 1. Figure out how many of these foods you consume every day, even more than once a day. Wheat, dairy, sugar, and yeast are the most common culprits.

Lab Tests

If your answers to the Food Intolerance Questionnaire indicate that a lab test should be your next step, then see Appendix II for more information.

Summary

There are a number of different methods for evaluating food intolerances. Most have some relevance and accuracy, but some do not. ELISA IgG analysis and the evaluation of chemical mediators, which also uses ELISA technology, are two of the most accurate and relevant tests.

Two different types of tests offering IgG analysis and analysis of the chemicals released in response to food antigen exposure are recommended. See Appendix II for more information.

Food intolerance testing is expensive, but can prove hugely useful in your mission to improve your health.

Part Two

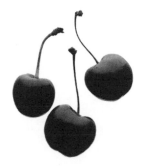

Why Do I Have a Food Intolerance?

3

Is It What I Eat?

Why Are Food Intolerances So Common?

This chapter will tell you about the reasons why food intolerances exist and why you may have one or more of them. You will find out how you can address your food intolerance and its underlying causes.

You have learned that at least 45 percent of the whole population has at least one food intolerance. Other researchers believe that this figure is as high as 80 percent. So why does this happen? Were we not designed to eat certain foods? Are more people intolerant to foods today than they were in the past?

First, let's review the most common causes of food intolerance. These causes may well be cumulative, may well co-exist and therefore may be synergistic in the cause of your food intolerance(s). Over the next few chapters we will look in detail at each of these causes.

- eating too much of the same food too often (this chapter)
- food additives, preservatives, coloring agents and flavor enhancers (this chapter)
- eating too quickly (Chapter 4)
- maldigestion (low stomach acid levels, low levels of pancreatic enzymes) (Chapter 4)
- imbalanced intestinal ecology: an overgrowth of yeast, bacteria or parasites (Chapters 5–7)
- prescription and over-the-counter drugs (Chapter 8)
- weak intestinal immunity and improved hygiene (Chapter 9)
- excess stress (Chapter 10).

The above list will have relevance to some people but not to others. For those of you for whom these factors are relevant, it is vital to address them in order to escape a vicious cycle involving food intolerances. I have had many patients tell me that they have followed an elimination diet to improve their symptoms. However, the reason they have come to see me is that, while the diet worked for a number of months, they ultimately ended up with the same symptoms, in spite of continuing to avoid the original culprit foods. Upon retesting we have learned that these patients were now suffering from new food intolerances. What is going on here is that the *underlying* causes are continuing to cause problems. In this way, food intolerance can be 'upstream' of a number of other problems – though it is worth bearing in mind that it can be 'downstream' as well.

This is the primary reason why you need to be aware of the associated and under-lying causes of food intolerance. To help you determine which of the seven most common causes of food intolerance may be relevant to you, each will be discussed in turn – where appropriate, questionnaires are provided to narrow down the potential culprits.

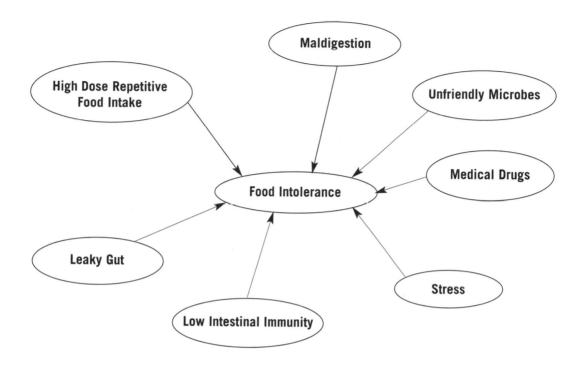

GI SYSTEM – Model of how food intolerance relates to other conditions

The diagram above shows the various factors that can contribute to food intolerance. Often there is more than one cause that you need to address.

Eating Too Much of the Same Food Too Often

Of the estimated 195,000 edible plants on the planet, we tend, in the Western world, to obtain most of our calories from fewer than 20 foods. Indeed, most people tend eat the same 10 foods every day (and this would most likely include wheat and dairy products). This predisposes you to having an altered immune reactivity to these foods. It also means that the variety of nutrients you derive from food will also be limited, which may have other effects on your health.

A simple seven-day food diary would highlight whether you are eating a predominance of only a handful of foods. Simply list the foods you eat every day for a whole week, and then check your list for the number of different food groups – for example, don't forget that most breakfast cereals, bread and pasta are all made from wheat. The higher the number of foods you eat in a typical week the better, and the more variety you have, the better. If you can identify that two or three foods comprise the bulk of your caloric intake, then these need to be suspected as possible culprits. You then have the option of eliminating these foods for a trial period and monitoring your symptoms.

You could also compare, as you may already have done, your typical food intake with the list of Usual Suspects (see pages 4–5), and especially the top five on that list.

Particularly if you have digestive symptoms, you should also follow the Digestive Support Plan for at least one month (see pages 154–6).

Food Additives, Preservatives, Coloring Agents and Flavor Enhancers

It is believed that the relatively recent plethora of food additives, colorings and preservatives in our diet has increased the risk of our immune system reacting against them, and this has been shown in at least one formal research study. It is also the subject of the Feingold Diet, which was named after Dr. Ben Feingold of San Francisco, who proposed that additives and other naturally-occurring chemicals in food cause hyperactivity and other problems in children.

The Feingold approach is well known in the nutritional arena. His approach of avoiding food additives can produce a dramatic difference in some children, and more moderate improvement in others. For example, the consumption of 'yellow sunset' coloring and tartrazine can have marked effects on some susceptible children's behavior, and therefore their avoidance can result in a total lack of such symptoms.

Feingold believed that the naturally-occurring chemicals in foods called salicylates, which are found in a wide array of foods, are also implicated in causing behavioral changes. However, it would appear that salicylates are not the lone culprit, because there are other offending agents at work, including solvent chemicals, that contribute to the children's symptoms.

Since food additives and preservatives are found primarily in pre-prepared foods, it should be fairly easy to spot when you might be consuming these artificial additives. However, even foodstuffs such as bread can contain additives. Therefore, anything that comes in packaging potentially has something artificial added to it. Start checking your labels and choose as much food as you can that is in its whole and natural state.

It is possible to test for an intolerance to additives – see Appendix II for more information.

A Note on Salicylates

This book does not provide you with salicylate-free recipes, but they are free of all additives, colorings and preservatives, and should contribute in a positive way to reducing your risk of adverse immune reactions within your gastro-intestinal tract. A list of foods containing salicylates is provided in Appendix V.

4

Digestive Difficulties

Eating Too Quickly

When you eat too quickly, food does not get chewed and broken down properly, so that when it reaches the stomach it is not in the ideal form for optimal digestion. This means the stomach acid and digestive enzymes are unable to digest this food, no matter what it is, and as a consequence intact proteins may be absorbed through the intestinal lining, setting up an immune reaction that can lead to the development of food intolerance. Eat more slowly and chew food thoroughly before swallowing it!

Chewing food well also helps stimulate protection within your intestinal lining, in the form of something called Epithelial Growth Factor (EGF). EGF helps support cell growth in the intestines. Chewing also lets your digestive system know that something is coming so that it can prepare itself, whereas scarfing your food can be a shock to your digestive system. Can you remember how many meals you have eaten in the past week when you chewed your food thoroughly?

When your mind is preoccupied while you are eating, your digestive system switches off. Your mind is giving your body the message that it is engaged in something, and this is not conducive to optimal digestion. Remember, if you cannot digest your food properly, it sets the scene for food intolerance. Typical examples are when you eat at your desk while working. Or eating while on the move. Or while watching TV. It is best to concentrate on the food you are eating to help your digestive system work at its best. The ritual of saying grace before a meal, for example, is an excellent means of setting the scene for your digestion. I'd encourage you all to 'give thanks' for the food you are about to eat, if only because it is one means by which you can improve your digestion.

CELIAC DISEASE

Celiac disease is another name for a gluten allergy (also called gluten-sensitive enteropathy) – which is *not* the same thing as a gluten intolerance. What happens in celiac disease is that the gluten proteins yield toxic fragments, or peptides, that damage the delicate cells of the intestinal lining. Over time, the surface area of the small intestine becomes damaged, causing a flattening or atrophy of the microvilli (tiny hairs that help with the transportation of food through the intestine). This leads to malabsorption of all nutrients (vitamins, minerals, fats, proteins, and carbohydrates) and, typically, weight loss, although many other conditions can ensue as well.

The reason this occurs is not wholly understood, but one theory is that there is a lack of appropriate digestive enzymes. Another theory is that the immune system perceives a part of the gluten protein to be 'foreign' and attacks it. In the ensuing battle, the immune system inadvertently damages the intestinal lining.

The symptoms include bloating, diarrhea, foul-smelling stools, pale stools, and poor growth in babies and children. In adults there can also be pain, malaise, weakness, and weight loss. Fatigue and irritability are also common. The skin and tongue may appear pale due to a lack of the normal red pigment found in blood. Bone problems may occur, such as deformity, pain, or propensity to fracture.

Since nutrients are incompletely absorbed, increased bowel frequency, with the passage of bulky, pale stools, may occur; there may be associated abdominal pain and/or distension. However, many sufferers experience no bowel disturbance, and may be constipated rather than suffer diarrhea.

It is likely that many people with gluten sensitivity have few or no symptoms, so the condition can remain unrecognized.

How Common Is It?
The condition affects approximately 1 in 1,000 people. If one family member is affected it is more likely that others in the same family will have it as well. The frequency of gluten sensitivity is greater than among the general population in people with certain other disorders, particularly those with the type of diabetes that requires insulin.

Although not backed by solid research evidence, one estimate puts the figure at much higher than 1 in a 1,000, and more like 1 in 200. This is consistent with the suggestion that for every celiac known there are five others who have yet to be identified. Perhaps with the wider recognition and acceptance of food intolerances, these individuals will either come forward or be identified by a doctor, and we will have a better idea of how widespread this problem is.

How Is It Treated?
Treatment involves avoiding all gluten foods – namely wheat, rye, barley, and oats.

Once the intestinal lining has been damaged, however, it can take some time to repair itself, and usually the individual needs to replenish nutrients either intravenously or orally. In many cases there are a host of other foods to which the celiac sufferer is intolerant (soy and milk, for instance) due to the damage done to the intestinal lining, which often means that even if they avoid gluten their health does not immediately return to normal.

What Complications Can Arise?

Women with untreated gluten sensitivity can experience infertility, though this reverses itself once glutens are withdrawn from the diet. Before and during pregnancy, women with gluten sensitivity should be particularly careful to take a supplement of folic acid, as advised for all women.

Thinning of bones (osteoporosis) may be more common among people with celiac disease than in the general population.

Dermatitis herpetiformis

People with an itchy, blistering skin eruption affecting the knees, elbows, buttocks and back, called dermatitis herpetiformis, almost always also show evidence of gluten sensitivity on intestinal biopsy. Zinc deficiency may also be a significant nutritionally-related issue with this condition, for which zinc supplements are needed.

Celiac Disease and Mental Health

Interestingly, many people with celiac disease also suffer bipolar disorder, highlighting the connection not only between the intestines and the brain but between gluten intolerance and brain functioning.

Symptoms associated with gluten intolerance (rather than celiac disease) include altered behavior, depression, irritability, and a short attention span.

An Inherited Disposition

It would appear that celiac disease is at least partly an inherited disposition, because it runs in families. It is a condition that does not have to be present at birth to later reveal itself. One belief is that celiac disease is a manifestation of humans' inability to adapt to wheat, which has only been available to humanity over the past 10,000 years – the blink of an eye in evolutionary terms. However, this does not explain the prevalence of wheat intolerance, the most likely cause of which is the sheer repetition and high doses that we consume, possibly at every meal and snack.

Celiac Testing

Just because you experience symptoms after eating foods that contain gluten, this does not mean you have celiac disease. The definitive test is a biopsy from the surface of the small intestine.

A flexible telescope (endoscope) is usually passed through the mouth into the stomach and upper intestine so that the lining can be inspected and a biopsy taken. This process takes only a few minutes and is often made easier and less uncomfortable by giving the patient a mild sedative beforehand. Alternatively, a biopsy can be obtained by swallowing a special capsule on the end of a narrow tube.

If the biopsy is abnormal, a second test may be advised after a period to check that the intestinal surface has returned to normal.

When there is doubt about an earlier diagnosis, or the changes seen on biopsy are uncertain, another biopsy may be advised after a person has deliberately eaten gluten for a period (this is called a 'gluten challenge').

Blood tests are helpful in detecting the body's reaction (antibodies) to gluten or as an indication of intestinal damage. The blood test that can give a strong indication of celiac disease analyzes tissue transglutaminase IgA levels along with reticulin and endomysial IgA antibodies. A positive result in this test also gives an indication of an inherited susceptibility to gluten intolerance. Other blood tests can be used to identify deficiencies of iron, vitamins such as folic acid, or minerals such as calcium. Such blood tests are useful for screening relatives or to ascertain whether a gluten sensitivity may be the cause of symptoms or of nutrient deficiency. These tests do not make the diagnosis, but indicate the advisability of a biopsy test.

If abdominal symptoms are troublesome or develop despite treatment, a barium X-ray of the intestine, which involves swallowing a tasteless white liquid, may be advised.

For more information about celiac disease, please contact:
American Celiac Society
c/o Annette Bentley
PO Box 23455
New Orleans, LA
70183
www.americanceliacsociety.org

Case Study: Digestion Is the Issue

Sarah Davies, 41, visited me in the summer a few years ago. She had been suffering from abdominal bloating and headaches for years. She was slim, which meant that whenever the bloating occurred, it was all the more obvious – this prevented her from going out in warm weather, it affected her so much. She found that eating most types of carbohydrates such as bread, pasta or potatoes triggered both the bloating and the headaches.

I recommended Sarah avoid the obvious culprit foods, which had the desired effect on her bloating and headaches. Trouble was, it meant that when she went out – and she had a very busy social life – she felt awkward not being able to eat those foods. Sarah also fulfilled the requirements for needing digestive enzymes. When she took these before and with food she could eat the culprit foods, once a day anyway, and get away with it both in terms of the bloating and the headaches. Needless to say, this transformed her life since she could now go out and not worry about what she ate.

Maldigestion

A lack of hydrochloric acid and pancreatic enzymes is a very common problem. If you cannot digest foods properly then there is an increased risk of food proteins crossing the intestinal lining, as well as an increased risk of intestinal permeability and transit time of food through the gastro-intestinal tract.

In addition to maldigestion, the lack of stomach acid can also represent a risk for the presence and survival of unwanted bacteria, yeast and parasites (more about this in later chapters).

Hydrochloric Acid (HCl)

HCl is the most acidic juice humans produce. Its main functions include:

- HCl secretion assists protein digestion by activating pepsinogen and turning it into pepsin
- HCl sterilizes the stomach against ingested pathogens (harmful bacteria, etc.)
- HCl prevents bacteria, yeast and fungi from growing in the small intestine
- HCl encourages the flow of bile
- HCl encourages the flow of pancreatic enzymes
- HCl facilitates the absorption of folic acid, vitamin B12, vitamins A and E, ascorbic acid, beta-carotene, non-heme iron and some forms of calcium, magnesium, and zinc.

Your body makes about 2 liters of gastric juices a day. In turn, the parietal cells produce HCl acid. HCl is produced in minimal amounts when you are not eating, at about 10 percent of maximal rate. The pH on an empty stomach should normally be about 1.8–2.0.

HOW DOES A LOW LEVEL OF STOMACH ACID AFFECT ME?

Low levels of stomach acid can lead to maldigestion of proteins, fats, and carbohydrates. Low HCl levels can lead to symptoms of indigestion: burping, abdominal bloating and excessive intestinal wind. It can lead to increased bacterial overgrowth in the small intestine as well as an increase in intestinal permeability (or leaky gut). Low HCl can also lead to the malabsorption of nutrients.

You should also be aware that the more protein you eat, the more HCl acid you need.

A COMMON PROBLEM

Low HCl levels are very common. The older you are, the more likely you are to have low levels. About 30 percent of the population over the age of 65 will be low in stomach acid (a condition known as hypochlorhydria).

There are a number of factors at work here, including stress and age. However, another is nutrient deficiency. Low levels of the mineral zinc and vitamins B1 and B6 can also play their part. Deficiencies in zinc and B vitamins are extremely common and are caused by not eating enough of the foods plentiful in these nutrients, to chronic stress (which increases our need for these nutrients) or to depleted levels caused by alcohol consumption or smoking.

HCl is responsible for vital digestive functions; if these cannot be carried out because your stomach acid levels are too low, you increase your risk of developing a food intolerance.

Your answers to the questionnaire (see page 6) will identify whether or not you should see your doctor for further advice. He or she will help you identify whether you should take HCl supplements.

A very small minority of people actually have high stomach acid levels, though their number is considerably lower than we are sometimes lead to believe.

BEWARE A BACTERIUM CALLED HELICOBACTOR PYLORI

If you do have low stomach acid levels, then you should also look to test for the presence of a bacterium called *Helicobacter pylori* before you start taking HCl supplements.

H. pylori is the most common chronic bacterial pathogen in humans. It lowers stomach acid levels while damaging the mucosal protection within the stomach. It has therefore been attributed with causing stomach and duodenal ulcers. If you took supplemental HCl while having *H. pylori* you would experience unpleasant side-effects, usually of a painful nature (sore, burning intestinal lining), which is why it is so important to rule out its presence before taking HCl. Ask your doctor for a breath test for *H. pylori*, because the blood test available cannot tell you whether you have successfully eradicated the bacterium.

If you do have *H. pylori* then follow the Anti-*H. pylori* Plan (see page 156), which lasts for six weeks. This is effective in about 80 to 90 percent of cases, which is as good as any antibiotic therapy, and will improve your symptoms more effectively than antibiotics. Two weeks after that, re-test for *H. pylori*. Finally, when you have eradicated the *H. pylori*, if your stomach acid levels are still low you can begin the Digestive Support Plan 2 (page 155).

Do I Have Low Stomach Acid?

Have you any of these symptoms? Score 1 for each 'yes' answer.

- bloating, belching, burning or wind immediately after eating
- indigestion
- dilated blood vessels in the cheeks and nose
- diarrhea or constipation
- iron deficiency
- itchy rectum
- nausea after taking supplements
- sense of fullness immediately after eating
- pimples, acne

- undigested food in stool
- persistent mucus in throat
- excess wind
- weak, peeling or cracked fingernails

In addition:
- Do you always eat in a rush?
- Do you not chew your food properly?

> Your score =   /15
>
> High Score = 5 (including two of the first three symptoms)
>   or 7 (not including the first two)

If you scored 5 or more, or answered 'yes' to two of the first three questions, then you should see your doctor to verify your stomach acid status. If you scored 7 or more and this did not include a 'yes' to any of the first three questions, you should nevertheless take the Gastro-Test. If you lack stomach acid then you should also rule out the presence of *H. pylori* before following Digestive Support Plan 2 (page 155). If you have *H. pylori*, you should follow the Anti-*H. pylori* Plan (page 156).

5

Digestive Enzymes, Yeasts and Parasites

Imbalanced Intestinal Ecology

The common expression 'you are what you eat' should more accurately be 'you are what you digest and absorb.' Even the most healthy foods will become toxic if you can't break them down properly.

Maldigestion of proteins, which are contained in most foods (not just high-protein foods), may be one of the most significant contributors to food intolerance. Some of the most common causes of maldigestion are the subject of this chapter.

Your pancreas is the major producer of digestive enzymes in the body – this accounts for over 90 percent of its function. Low levels of the pancreatic enzymes required to digest food are remarkably common, as identified by lab tests. However, this deficiency state does not mean that everyone has clinical signs of fat-malabsorption syndrome – the conventional assessment of pancreatic enzyme output. Rather, chronic pancreatic enzyme insufficiency (chronically low levels of pancreatic enzymes) may contribute to a wide variety of health problems well before this condition manifests.

The most likely causes of this are stress, eating too quickly, and even low stomach acid levels. If you have a low output of pancreatic enzymes, then you may suffer from maldigestion with an increased risk of malabsorption. This means that improperly digested food can sit in the intestine and provide nourishment for unwanted bacteria. As they consume what you cannot digest, this causes increased fermentation of the food and, as gases are released, excess wind.

Whether or not you are inadvertently feeding unwelcome guests in your intestine, the incomplete breakdown of proteins in what you eat is highly likely to increase inappropriate immunological activity in the intestine, with an increased risk of food intolerance. This also has the knock-on effect of increasing intestinal permeability, discussed more fully in Chapter 11, which allows larger proteins to cross the intestinal lining and enter the bloodstream. There they act as antigens, to which the body makes antibodies, and this often causes symptoms. Even trace amounts of undigested protein absorbed into the blood can cause profound reactions.

Supplements

Taking digestive enzymes in supplement form has been found to alleviate the symptoms of wheat sensitivity because they help the body digest the proteins in wheat (probably gliadin in the gluten fraction of wheat). Even as long ago as the 1940s, supplements of hydrochloric acid and pancreatic enzymes were used to treat digestive and allergic-type conditions such as asthma and eczema. This is why digestive enzymes, such as Bio 6 Plus, are part of the Digestive Support Plan (see pages 154–6) recommended for anyone who wants to improve their digestive health and reduce the impact of food intolerances in their lives.

Do Supplemental Digestive Enzymes Survive Stomach Acid?

The answer is *Yes*. In addition to much clinical evidence, there is much peer-reviewed evidence to support this (see References for this chapter, page 317). This is particularly true of animal-source enzymes chymotrypsin and trypsin, which have found to be more helpful in supporting digestion than plant enzymes such as bromelain and papain.

Should I Drink with Meals or Not?

Fluids consumed with meals actually help to *stimulate* stomach acid and digestive enzymes in the small intestine. In fact, sufficient fluid with a meal is essential for an optimal response from your digestive system.

How Can I Tell If I Have Low Levels of Digestive Enzymes?

The signs and symptoms of a lack of digestive enzymes present us with yet another list of overlapping symptoms which could ultimately relate to almost any condition in the body related to malnourishment or food intolerance. Therefore, only the major signs and symptoms are included in the questionnaire below. Since digestive enzymes are recommended to one and all in the Digestive Support Plans (beginning on page 154), this next questionnaire should be used primarily as an aid to monitoring your improvement.

Score 1 point for each 'yes' answer.

Do you regularly suffer from any of the following?

- abdominal bloating or swelling

- wind after meals

- undigested food in the stool

- signs of poor digestion of fatty foods

- weak, peeling or cracked fingernails

- any skin condition

- recurring headaches

- depression

- fatigue in spite of a good diet and regular sleep

- inability to gain muscle despite regular weight training

In addition:

- Do you always eat in a rush?

- Do you not chew your food properly?

Your score =   /12

High Score =   7 or more

If you scored 4 or more, then you should take Bio 6 Plus as detailed in the Digestive Support Plan (pages 154–6). If you scored 5 or 6, take two of Bio 6 Plus tablets with each meal, then review your score for stomach acid levels (questionnaire, pages 55–6). If you scored 7 or more, take three Bio 6 tablets before or at each meal, review your need for stomach acid as outlined above, and observe whether this improves your symptoms.

Relevant Tests: Stool Analysis (Comprehensive Stool Analysis)

Since a stool analysis is not the most accurate method of identifying digestive enzyme output, if you score highly you should take digestive enzymes and observe your symptoms first, before undertaking a stool test.

6

How Healthy Is My
Intestinal Ecology?

The intestinal lining is coated with and contains over 400 different species of micro-organisms, or intestinal flora – both healthful and unhealthful bacteria numbering in the billions. One estimate is that the bacteria in your colon weigh 3 lb, and that the number of individual bacteria outnumbers the number of human cells in your body.

Intestinal bacteria carry out so many functions in the body that they can almost be considered an organ in their own right. We truly have a symbiotic relationship with our intestinal microflora. The balance of these bacteria plays a vital role in determining intestinal health; they are a front-line immune defence, and when in optimal balance help to control absorption, the production of nutrients, the level of toxins and the elimination of unwanted matter.

Do I Need More Probiotics?

Probiotics is a word used to describe micro-organisms that work against disease-causing microbes (i.e. pathogens). Probiotic organisms can have a significant influence on the treatment and prevention of disease. They can even influence blood cholesterol levels.

The famous Russian Nobel Prize Winner, Elie Metchnikoff (1845–1916) identified that the long lifespan of the Bulgarians was due to the probiotics in their habitual *kefir* drink. One strain of probiotic – *Lactobacillus bulgaricus* – has been named after them. Metchnikoff attributed so much importance to our intestinal bacteria that he has been quoted as saying, 'Death begins in the colon.'

How Can Probiotics Help Me?

There is increasing evidence that imbalanced bacteria levels in the intestine – known as *dysbiosis* – is a cause or contributory factor in Chronic Fatigue Syndrome, Irritable Bowel Syndrome (IBS), arthritic conditions, and depression. In fact, in one well-conducted study, 16 out of 20 long-term sufferers of diarrhea were cured with the use of probiotics.

Probiotic agents have a wide array of actions:

- They help produce anti-microbial substances.
- They help stop the growth of unwanted pathogenic bacteria.
- They help keep unwanted bacteria from sticking to your intestinal lining.
- They stimulate local and peripheral immunity.
- They stimulate the production of enzymes made by the intestinal lining itself (called 'brush-border enzymes').
- They stimulate SIgA (Secretory Immunoglobulin A, secreted by the intestinal lining).

- They help stop bacteria from leaving the intestine and getting into the blood-stream.

It is likely that probiotics prevent unwanted bacteria from colonizing your intestines through direct suppression of harmful micro-organisms and the stimulation of beneficial organisms.

There are many beneficial strains of probiotics, with *Lactobacillus acidophilus* and *Lactobacillus casei* demonstrating the ability to activate the immune system. Do bear in mind that you should only take supplements that have earned scientific backing.

Why Should I Take Probiotics?

Unfortunately, there are many bad habits which can upset the delicate balance of flora in the intestines. A diet high in refined carbohydrates (e.g. white flour and sugar), processed and refined foods, and fried and high-fat foods (e.g. fast foods) all contribute to feeding the wrong kind of bacteria and would also support the proliferation of yeast and fungi. This type of diet is also associated with less frequent bowel motions and other chronic digestive conditions. Excess alcohol is certainly harmful, as is the use of antacids (see page 82).

When you need to restore probiotic levels or use them for a therapeutic purpose, it is not as simple as taking one product indefinitely. In fact, the high-dose probiotics may not be necessary long term when low-dose (and cheaper) probiotics can serve the purpose. It is best to use a single strain or limited number of strains in high strength for the first few weeks, after which a mixed-strain formula should be used. Then, for maintenance, a low-dose probiotic of a different strain again should be used. This is the approach implemented in the supplement plans detailed in Part 3.

A Probiotic Yeast?

If you suffer from an overgrowth of the yeast *Candida albicans* (normally present in the bowel, and causing no problems unless it is allowed to over-run), there are two strains of probiotic yeast that can help. One is made by Allergy Research and is called *Saccharomyces boulardii*; the other is made by BioCodex and is sold under the name Florastor. These probiotic yeasts work by binding to the Candida yeast and thus keeping it in check and supporting your overall intestinal immunity.

Have I Got a Yeast Overgrowth?

A study was undertaken to see how well the results of this questionnaire compared to stool analysis for the presence of *Candida albicans*. The degree of *Candida albicans* growth on stool culture correlated well with the symptom scores revealed by the questionnaire.

Culture Results (average values)	Questionnaire Results
No growth	49.5
1–2 colonies	67
3–6 colonies	97.9
7–11 colonies	113.3
12+ colonies	117.9

This questionnaire will be helpful for finding out whether you should undergo a test to prove the existence of yeast overgrowth.

Yeast Overgrowth

Filling out and scoring this questionnaire should help you and your practitioner evaluate the possible role of Candida in contributing to your health problem.

This questionnaire was designed by William Crook for adults; the scoring system is not appropriate for children. It addresses factors in your medical history (Section A) as well as the symptoms commonly found in individuals with yeast-connected illness (Sections B and C).

For each 'Yes' answer in Section A, circle the Point Score in that section. Total your score and record it at the end of the section. Then move on to Sections B and C and score as directed.

Section A: History

1. Have you taken tetracycline (or other antibiotics) for 2 months (or longer)?   25
2. Have you, at any time in your life, taken other 'broad-spectrum' antibiotics (including Keflex®, ampicillin, amoxicillin, Ceclor®, Bactrim®, and Septra®*) for respiratory, urinary or other infections for two months or longer, or in shorter courses four or more times in a one-year period?   20
3. Have you, at any time in your life, been troubled by persistent vaginal problems or had three or more episodes of vaginitis in a year?   25

4. Have you been pregnant more than twice?   5
   Have you been pregnant once?   3
5. Have you taken birth control pills for more than two years?   15
   For six months to two years?   18
6. Have you taken prednisone, Decadron® or other cortisone-type
   drugs for more than two weeks?   15
   For less than two weeks?   6
7. Does exposure to perfumes, insecticides, fabric-shop odours and
   other chemicals provoke ...
   Moderate to severe symptoms?   20
   Mild symptoms?   5
8. Are your symptoms worse on damp, muggy days or in moldy places? 20
9. Have you had persistent athlete's foot, 'jock itch' or other chronic
   fungal infections of the skin or nails? Have such infections been ...
   Severe or persistent?   20
   Mild to moderate?   10
10. Do you crave sugar?   10
11. Do you crave breads?   10
12. Do you crave alcohol?   10
13. Does tobacco smoke really bother you?   10

Total Section A =

Section B: Major Symptoms

For each symptom present, enter the appropriate number of points in the Point Score column:

> If a symptom is mild, score 3 points
>
> If a symptom is moderate, score 6 points
>
> If a symptom is severe or disabling, score 9 points

Point Score

1. fatigue or lethargy
2. feeling of being 'drained'
3. poor memory
4. feeling 'spacey' or 'unreal'
5. depression
6. numbness, burning or tingling
7. muscle aches
8. muscle weakness or paralysis
9. pain and/or swelling in joints
10. abdominal pain
11. constipation
12. diarrhea
13. bloating
14. troublesome vaginal discharge
15. persistent vaginal burning or itching
16. prostatitis (inflamed, enlarged prostate)
17. impotence
18. loss of sexual feeling
19. endometriosis
20. dysmenorrhea (painful periods)
21. premenstrual tension

22. spots in front of eyes

23. erratic vision

Total Score Section B =

Section C: Other Symptoms

For each symptom which is present, enter the appropriate number of points in the Point Score column:

> If a symptom is mild, score 1 point
>
> If a symptom is moderate, score 2 points
>
> If a symptom is severe or disabling, score 3 points

While the symptoms in this section occur commonly in patients with yeast-connected illness, they also occur commonly in patients who do not have an overgrowth of Candida.

Point Score

1. drowsiness

2. irritability or jitteriness

3. lack of co-ordination

4. inability to concentrate

5. frequent mood swings

6. headache

7. dizziness/loss of balance

8. pressure above the ears/feeling as though your head is swelling and/or tingling

9. itching

10. rashes

11. heartburn

12. indigestion

13. belching and intestinal gas

14. mucus in stools

15. hemorrhoids

16. dry mouth

17. blisters or a rash in mouth

18. bad breath

19. joint swelling or arthritis

20. nasal congestion or discharge

21. post-nasal drip

22. nasal itching

23. sore or dry throat

24. cough

25. pain or tightness in chest

26. wheezing or shortness of breath

27. urinary urgency or frequency

28. burning on urination

29. failing vision

30. burning or tearing eyes

31. recurrent ear infections

32. fluid in ears

33. ear pain or deafness

34. history of grommets

35. Other symptoms:

Total Score, Section C =

> Section A   . . . .
> Section B   . . . .
> Section C   . . . .
> **Total**   . . . .

Evaluating Your Score

Note that the scoring will be different for men and women, since seven questions apply exclusively to women, while only two apply exclusively to men.

Over 180 (women)/140 (men)	Candida almost certainly plays a role in causing your health problems
Over 120 (women)/90 (men)	Candida probably plays a role in causing your health problems
60–120 (women)/40–90 (men)	Candida possibly plays a role in causing your health problems
Less than 60 (women)/40 (men)	Candida is less apt to be playing a significant role in causing your health problems

Interpretation

If you have scored over 120 (women) or 90 (men) BUT you do NOT score highly in any of the other questionnaires in this book – and have therefore not been instructed to take any tests other than a Food Intolerance test – then you should undertake a Candida Antibody test.

If positive, then you should follow the Anti-Yeast Plan and additional dietary recommendations (see pages 156–7).

> **Relevant Tests: Yeast Culture**

7

'Uninvited Guests'

Parasites – 'UFOs of the Intestines'

Once considered to be a sign of the unclean, 'uncivilized' and unhygienic in faraway lands, intestinal parasites are much closer to home that you'd think. The prevalence of previously unidentified fecal organisms (UFOs) is staggeringly high. According to most parasitology specialists, 40 percent of the world's population are infected by one parasite or another. Anne Louise Gittelman, author of *Guess What Came to Dinner?*, estimates that parasites are present in even greater numbers, with eight out of ten people being affected. Laboratory evidence supports the claims of the former. Parascope, based in the U.K., finds that 40 percent of specimens contain parasites. In the US, one of the most accurate labs for this sort of assessment, the Doctors' Data Lab, find parasites in 20 percent of samples tested. It should be noted that these labs are capable of great accuracy when testing for parasites. The Centers for Disease Control in Atlanta found that one out of six randomly selected people had one or more parasites. Over 130 different types of parasites have been found in Americans. Just a few years ago, the incidence of *Blastocystis hominis* infection in the US was up to 12 percent, while in tropical countries this figure ranges from 20 to 50 percent.

Even if we accept the lowest estimates, we are still left with a huge number of people carrying parasites. Dr. Hermann Bueno is one of the world's most experienced parasitologists, and he believes that 'Parasites are the missing diagnosis in the genesis of many chronic health problems, including diseases of the gastrointestinal tract and endocrine system.'

One of the reasons why this may not be fully appreciated is that the usual and conventional methods of determining the presence of parasites is not accurate. Many U.K. laboratories do not use techniques that can help identify parasites. In 1976 a U.K. study published in the *Lancet* showed that the average adult with the parasite *Giardia lamblia* needed an average of 16 consecutive investigations before the infection was diagnosed. Other studies have shown that organisms which have long been thought to be harmless residents of the intestinal tract can in fact cause ill health.

Just from my own clinical experience, it is often the case that by using a lab with accurate testing methods, these uninvited guests are identified where they have not been unearthed by hospital tests. On one occasion, three parasites were identified in one client who had been suffering from Chronic Fatigue, after six – yes, six – hospital tests had failed to pick this up.

How Did I Pick Up UFOs?

The major sources of contamination are from tap water, improperly cooked or stored food, pets and their feces, human feces (from diapers, etc.) and via infections acquired abroad. The international spread of parasitic infections has occurred relatively swiftly and is due, at least in part, to the very same causes behind the rise of food intolerances.

International travel should not be played down in its role as a source of parasitic infection. For example, I will never forget that when I visited St. Petersburg in 1989 there was a *Giardia* infection in the whole of the city's water supply. We were advised that bottled water was a must, even for brushing our teeth.

Filarial worms, hookworms, whipworms, pinworms, flatworms, and ameba affect more than two billion people around the world, not just confined to the developing world, causing a long list of afflictions ranging from elephantitis to blindness and serious intestinal problems. They are also potentially one of the biggest causes of food intolerance.

It matters not whether you are rich or poor. Parasites attack all socio-economic groups, including movie stars and the families of reputable cardiac surgeons.

Who's Who of UFOs

The most common parasites are:

Blastocystis hominis

Dientameba fragilis

Entameba coli

Giardia lamblia

Endolimax nana

Cryptosporidium

The Signs and Symptoms of UFO Infection

When the body is inhabited or colonized by unwanted bacteria, excess yeast, or parasites for more than just short episodes, this reflects an imbalance not only within the digestive tract but also with the immune system. Weakened immunity significantly increases the risk of infection by these unwanted organisms, and parasites are no exception. In this way, the scene that favors food intolerances is also one that favors parasites.

In fact, food intolerance is a possible sign of parasite infection, and the symptoms can be similar. It is believed that parasites alter immune activity in the intestine and increase inflammation – both of which increase the risk of immunoglobulin G reactivity to food antigens. The direct association between parasites and food intolerances is something of gray area in terms of diagnosis, but there are some solid links. The inflammation caused by parasites and the toxins they produce can also increase the risk of leaky gut syndrome, and it is this that most certainly leads to food intolerance. In this way, there may be a strong indirect association between parasitic infection and food intolerance, and a possible direct link, too. Check out the list and see if you are a contender for hosting a UFO.

Have I Got Parasites?

Score 1 point for each of these questions.

Do any of the following regularly apply to you?

1. anemia
2. excess wind
3. bloating
4. abdominal fullness
5. nausea

6. constipation

7. diarrhea or irregular bowel motions

8. abdominal cramps or pain

9. fatigue

10. unexplained fevers

11. Inflammatory Bowel Disease (IBS) such as colitis or Crohn's Disease

12. hives

13. teeth-grinding

14. weight loss (unexplained by any change in diet)

15. rectal bleeding

16. joint and/or muscle aches and pains

17. food intolerances

18. owning pets

19. having children who visit other children who have pets

20. frequent international travel

21. drinking only tap water

22. history of previous parasitic infections (even if treated)

23. history of traveler's diarrhea

24. history of family members with parasites

25. difficulty overcoming intestinal yeast growth

Your Score =   /25

High Score = 15 or more

Interpretation

The questionnaire does not diagnose parasites, rather it highlights the possibility that parasites are present. Therefore, a high score is suggestive of a need to consider a test to identify them. If parasites exist, then it may prove to be very important to address them and not just any food intolerance issues, especially as they may contribute to an ongoing risk of food intolerance to any foods you consume regularly.

0–5	You need not undergo a test for the presence of parasites. Continue to implement the plan most appropriate for you (see Part 3), but if you meet with no success then reconsider this section along with your responses to the other questionnaires in the book, and try following the parasite prevention program as described in Part 3 as well as the Digestive Support Plan.
6–9	Already, you are scoring too high for comfort and it raises the possibility of an unwanted bug within your digestive tract. Since many of the symptoms overlap with other possible imbalances, however, you need to put this result into the correct context. It may transpire that you are already being advised to undertake a stool test for something else; this could reveal more information about possible parasites. Follow the parasite prevention programme as described in Part 3, as well as the Digestive Support Plan.
10–14	You should do the Comprehensive Parasitology Test IF, after four weeks, dietary changes relating to food intolerance (including the Digestive Support Plan) do NOT improve your score to below 10.
15 or more	The higher your score above 15, the more important it is to rule out the presence of parasites with the stool analysis called Comprehensive Parasitology. This test also examines for yeasts and bacteria. Arrange the test via the lab and implement the dietary changes and Digestive Support Plan outlined for you with regard to food intolerances once you have sent the samples off.

Case Study: Parasites Prove to Be a Key

Michael Jones, 21, had a long-term fatigue condition but also had digestive complaints including bloating, excessive wind and irregular bowel, resembling Irritable Bowel Syndrome. Interestingly, this had come along only in the past six months, whereas he had been inappropriately fatigued for a few years. A food intolerance test identified his culprit foods, which he avoided. His digestive symptoms were 75 percent improved. Next, a stool test identified the presence of a parasite; this was addressed by nutritional means. After a matter of a few weeks, he found that he could eat the foods he was 'intolerant' to and not experience unpleasant symptoms. The improvement lasted both during and after the Anti-parasite Plan.

Relevant Tests: Stool Analysis (Comprehensive Parasitology)

The best method of testing for parasites is with a stool sample, or two, which are analyzed by powerful microscopy. This should be accompanied by appropriate antibody testing, which means the lab also looks for whether your body is making antibodies to the bugs. This increases the tests' accuracy by about 40 percent. The test that Doctor's Data offer is one of the best and most accurate in the world (see Appendix III).

A Note about Unwelcome Bacteria

Since the signs and symptoms of unwelcome bacteria such as *Proteus* species, *Klebsiella pneumoniae*, *Citrobacter freundii* and *Pseudomonas aeruginosa* are identical to those of parasites or yeast overgrowth, there is no specific questionnaire to help identify the presence of these. Your answers to the yeast and parasite questionnaires should give you the course of action that will help you address these.

8

Prescription and
Over-the-Counter Drugs

Antibiotics

Since antibiotics alter the bowel bacteria and inhibit probiotics, they can affect functions within the intestinal lining, lowering intestinal immunity and paving the way for the growth of unwanted bacteria. These can further deplete intestinal immunity and increase the risk of leaky gut syndrome. It is unlikely that one single course of antibiotics will cause too much trouble, but repeated courses almost certainly will cause some digestive imbalance or other. If antibiotics are given to babies or young children this can also set the scene for adverse reactions to foods. This is especially true if the antibiotic is given for the wrong reason or for too long a period of time. For example, glue ear is almost always caused by a negative reaction to cow's milk products but antibiotics are often prescribed repeatedly. This diminishes the friendly bacteria and further increases the likelihood that the young child will develop other intolerances.

Antibiotics are also well known for permitting the growth of yeast in the colon. This is because antibiotics inhibit the growth of bacteria but do not have any impact on yeast, which is a different kind of microbe. This is the time when probiotics and in particular *Saccharomyces boulardii* should be prescribed (see page 65).

It is also not uncommon for individuals actually to have an intolerance or allergy to antibiotics. These can also be tested for.

.

The Contraceptive Pill

There is also clinical evidence, though admittedly no strong study, to support the idea that the contraceptive Pill can cause food intolerances. This may be due to the fact that the hormones in the Pill affect certain liver-detoxification enzymes, thereby making a woman more susceptible to the negative effects of toxins in foods and from the environment. The Pill also depletes vitamins (B vitamins, vitamin A) and minerals (zinc, magnesium, manganese, and iron) and tends to increase copper levels.

There is also statistical evidence that the Pill increases the chance of a yeast overgrowth.

Combine antibiotics and the Pill and there may be a synergistic negative effect within the intestine, thereby increasing the risk not only of food intolerance but also of yeast overgrowth.

Steroids

Steroids suppress intestinal immunity and thereby increase the risk of unwanted microbes setting up home, as well as the direct risk of food intolerance due to decreased SIgA (more about this in Chapter 9). Long-term use of steroids such as prednisone, also increases the risk of altered intestinal permeability due to the suppressive effect that the steroid has on protein turnover in the body.

NSAIDs

Non-steroidal anti-inflammatory drugs (NSAIDs) such as aspirin and ibuprofen are well known for causing tissue damage in the intestinal lining. Microscopy photographs of the stomach lining taken before and then 16 minutes after the ingestion of 150 mg of aspirin reveal lesions in the stomach wall that can be seen quite clearly. As is well known, NSAIDs remain one of the main causes of gastric ulcers.

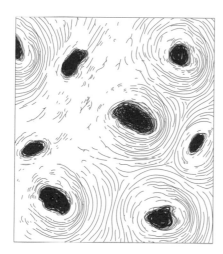 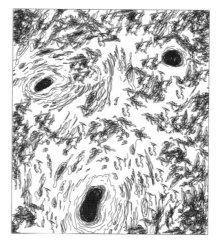

NSAID damage to the gastric mucosa
Scanning electron micrographs of normal gastric mucosa (left) and
mucosa surface (right) 16 minutes after administration of aspirin

Antacids

Antacids are the most commonly doctor-prescribed and self-prescribed over-the-counter medicines used to counteract indigestion, acid reflux, hiatal hernia, and heartburn. Long-term use of antacids actually increases the risk of food intolerance, in spite of the fact that the symptoms for which people take antacids are often caused by food intolerance in the first place.

9

Intestinal Immunity

Secretory Immunoglobulin A (SIgA) is the most abundant immune protein in the whole body; its reactions are non-inflammatory. It coats the mucosal surfaces in your body, the largest of which is your intestinal lining. It is designed to protect us from the inside. However, low levels can increase the risk of inflammatory immune reactions to proteins and undigested food molecules. Low levels increase the risk of leaky gut syndrome and of the adherence and growth of unfriendly microbes in the intestinal lining.

SIgA is by no means the only immune cell in the intestines, which are saturated with immune defenses. However, it is their front-line defense.

Many of the causes of food intolerance – including stress, some drugs, and imbalanced intestinal ecology – can directly lower SIgA levels. There are a number of direct and indirect means by which you can either prevent the suppression of SIgA or actually increase its output. An almost certain way to increase SIgA is to follow the SIgA Plan as detailed in Part 3.

It is also fair to note here that most experts believe that the increase in food intolerances and other allergies may also be related to the improved hygiene that we have in society today. By failing to expose ourselves to substances that might provoke the production of antibodies (i.e. antigenic material), we fail to stimulate our intestinal immunity. As a result, white blood cells which would normally become T Cells of one type actually become T Cells of another type entirely, and which are capable of producing inflammatory messengers called cytokines (e.g. TNF-a). Taking probiotics may be able to reduce the expression of such cells and thereby reduce inflammation.

You should only undertake a SIgA test if you score high on the questionnaire in the next chapter BUT have NOT scored high in any other questionnaire, including The Food Intolerance Questionnaire.

> **Relevant Tests: SIgA**

Summary

Although you may find, like Sally Ann (see Introduction) that it's a single food that is causing your symptoms, it is actually more likely that there are a number of factors involved. And the longer you have been troubled by your intolerance, the more likely this is.

In this chapter you have seen what the major causes for food intolerance are (aside from stress, which is the subject of the next chapter), and have been presented with the four questionnaires that will help you to identify how best to address specific digestive issues.

The specific Action Plans you will need to follow are presented in Part 3.

At least 50 percent of people with food intolerances have at least one other distinct problem as well. As the model on page 43 shows, there are many potential associated conditions with food intolerance.

This book will help you build up a comprehensive picture of how your food intolerances are affecting your health and be able to identify and improve all of your associated symptoms.

10

The Stress Factor

This chapter focuses on the emotional and stress-related aspects of digestive function.

There is a well-known link between stress and Irritable Bowel Syndrome (IBS), and a very strong link between IBS and food intolerance. In 1982, a paper in the *Lancet* highlighted that the major factor in the development of IBS was indeed food intolerance. It is also known that excess stress causes a reduction in SIgA (Secretory Immunoglobulin A – see page 104), which in turn increases the risk of food intolerance. More importantly, stress has a direct effect on the digestive system.

Does IBS Cause Stress?

Yes, IBS can actually be a cause of stress, as well as the other way round. The research supports this strongly. What happens follows two main pathways. For example, inflammation caused by food intolerances or dysbiosis within the digestive system produces many different chemicals which are the mediators of that inflammation. These chemicals can enter the bloodstream or become the subject of immune-defense reactions in the body, resulting in immune complexes. These immune complexes travel in the bloodstream and are perceived by the brain, and in particular by the hypothalamus. The hypothalamus gland controls much of the work of the pituitary gland – the master gland or conductor of the body's hormonal orchestra.

When the hypothalamus perceives the markers of inflammation, it responds by producing anti-inflammatory hormones. These hormones are produced by your adrenal glands, which sit on your kidneys. The major hormone produced is cortisol. In this way, the inflammatory discomfort in your intestines stimulates a gland in your brain to send a message to the adrenals to produce more stress hormones. If this only happens now and again, it will not have any deleterious effects on your body. However, if this happens repeatedly it can lead to 'exstressive' responses – that is, the body's normal stress response is triggered too easily and too often. Especially when combined with the rest of life's stressors, the pain in your intestines also increases the risk of adrenal fatigue – a very real problem that is largely misunderstood by the medical world, which tends to believe that the adrenal glands are in perfect working order unless you have Cushing's Disease (overactive adrenal glands) or Addison's Disease (underactive adrenal glands). Furthermore, an elevated level of cortisol diminishes SIgA levels and impedes repair of your intestinal lining.

As if this were not enough, the second main mechanism by which IBS causes stress is via the immediate nerve stimulation from within the intestines. The intestines have been referred to as 'man's second brain' – not least because they contain a tremendous number of nerves which both receive and impart information and messages. If there is discomfort in the stomach or intestines, then in a matter of split-seconds your central nervous system will know about it. This puts your body into 'sympathetic mode', which is the same mode as if you were under duress, preparing your body for fight or flight. This 'alert' mode decreases blood supply to your digestive system and shunts more to your large muscles. The lack of blood flow to your digestive functions can readily exacerbate digestive problems, creating a vicious cycle. In this way, once IBS has been established for some time, stress has an impact from two perspectives – external forces (the stresses of life) and internal ones. In most cases, support for both works best.

The questionnaire below will help you to establish the level of lifestyle stress that may have an impact on your digestive system.

Have I Got Stress-related Digestive Problems?

For each 'yes' answer, score 1 point.

1. **Are you busy all the time?** – This keeps your brain stimulating cortisol, a prime adrenal hormone that keeps the body in 'sympathetic' stress mode. In excess levels this not only lowers SIgA but also diminishes protein-turnover and healing, which are vital for the intestinal lining, normally one of the most rapidly-repairing tissues in the body.
2. **Do you feel frustrated all the time?** – This emotional state lowers SIgA more profoundly than any other.
3. **Are you chronically or constantly anxious?** – Even low-grade anxiety raises cortisol, and some of us do not even recognize this until we go on vacation and crash when we have nothing to do! This has a similar but less profound effect on your SIgA than frustration.
4. **Do you eat too quickly?** – So fast that food barely touches the sides? Your

stomach has no teeth, so it is always best to chew food thoroughly before swallowing. This can be a habit that dies hard. Undigested or poorly-digested food challenges your intestinal immunity and increases the risk of non-SIgA reactions. Slow down and chew your food well.

5. Do you experience abdominal bloating within 30 minutes of eating? – Bloating this soon after eating reveals that you are not digesting food properly or that there is a lack of 'energy' within your digestive system. It may also be a food intolerance reaction. Again, slow down and chew your food well.

6. Do you suffer frequent indigestion or burping or excess wind after meals? – Especially when you are in a rush? This reflects low stomach acid, one of the risks of food intolerance. Once again, slow down and chew your food well.

7. Do you have cravings for salt, salty foods, or sugar? – Do you find yourself eating the whole bag of chips or adding extra salt to foods, and/or you craving sugar or something sweet on a regular basis? This is a reflection of adrenal stress and an indirect measure of how stress might be involved in your overall health.

8. Do you experience an 'energy crash' after eating a moderate-sized meal? – This can often be the case especially after lunch: Even though you have not eaten a large meal, you find that a normal meal makes you want to take a nap afterwards. This is a sign of adrenal fatigue, and could also be a sign of food intolerance itself.

9. Do your symptoms get worse if you skip meals or eat too little? – Do you have to drive yourself with snacks, colas, and coffees just to keep from collapsing? This is a measure of stress that is indirectly related to your digestive health.

10. Are you constantly tired even though you are getting enough sleep? – Despite getting a good night's sleep, do you still feel tired when you wake up?

'Refreshed' is a foreign word to people with adrenal fatigue. This reflects that your digestive system does not have enough energy to digest food properly.

11. **Are you lethargic?** – Does everything seem like a chore, even the things you used to enjoy? This reflects that your digestive system does not have enough energy to digest food properly.

12. **Do you tire easily and have no stamina?** – Does everything take more effort? If walking a block sometimes feels like a marathon, this reflects that your digestive system does not have enough energy to digest food properly.

13. **Do you have difficulty handling stress?** – Do little things that never used to bother you, now get to you? Anger, road rage, constant anxiety, yelling at your kids, compulsive eating, smoking or drug use are some of the behaviors that let you know your adrenals are crying out for help. This reflects that your digestive system does not have enough energy to digest food properly.

14. **Does it take you a long time to recover from illness, injury or trauma?** – The cold you got in October is still hanging on in December. The cut on your finger takes weeks to heal. Two years after your father died you are still incapacitated by grief. Slow wound-healing directly impacts on the healing of your intestinal lining.

15. **Have your PMS symptoms increased?** – Bloated, tired, crabby, crampy and craving chocolate – does it get any worse than this? This usually means that your digestive system does not have enough energy to digest food properly, and also that refined carbohydrates and sugar may be feeding unwanted bacteria and yeast in your intestines.

16. **Do you feel light-headed if you stand up too quickly?** – If you sometimes feel a little woozy or even like you are going to pass out when you get up too quickly from the bed or a chair, this is a sign of adrenal fatigue, which has an impact on your digestive system's ability to work properly.

17. **Do you find it difficult getting up in the morning?** – Three alarms and you

still don't feel awake enough to lift your head off the pillow. This is another sign of adrenal fatigue which has an indirect effect on your digestion and immune functions.

18. **Do you hit an afternoon 'low' between 3 and 4 p.m.?** – At around 3.00–3.30 in the afternoon you start to feel like you have been drugged, and this is usually the time you reach for chocolate or a sugary snack. This reflects two things: that you have adrenal fatigue (and this influences digestive energies) and that you are feeding your intestines the wrong food.

19. **Have you lost muscle tone?** – If despite the same levels of activity you appear to have less muscle relative to body weight, this reflects that your body may not be healing and repairing itself as well as it should – and this will affect your intestinal lining before it affects your muscles.

20. **Have you got high blood pressure?** – Stress raises blood pressure by a number of mechanisms including elevated cortisol levels. Stress also inhibits digestive functions.

21. **Do you suffer from insomnia?** – This is one of the classic signs of stress. Cortisol at high levels is a direct cause of interrupted sleep. This can directly affect immunity in the intestines and the rate at which the intestinal lining repairs itself.

22. **Do you exercise too much?** – Are you exercising six or more times a week for more than 45 minutes at a time, or for more than 90 minutes four or more times a week? This is a classic cause of low SIgA. Please note that you are more likely to experience a food intolerance reaction after intense or endurance exercise than at other times. This is why it is useful to use appropriate sports powders after exercise sessions so that you can replace lost energy with easy-to-digest carbohydrates rather than something like pasta.

23. **Are you overly competitive?** – Regularly participating in competitive sport will increase your levels of 'anticipatory' (before-the-event) stress as well as your

levels of performance stress. Most athletes need to do something to support their SIgA levels (see point 22).

24. **Do you suffer from chronic pain?** – No matter what the source, this leads to excess cortisol stimulation. This has the same effect as excess stress and lowers intestinal immunity and increases the risk of leaky gut syndrome.

25. **Are you drinking too much?** – Do you drink more than three glasses of alcohol more than twice a week? Alcohol impairs the liver's ability to use glycogen for brain sugar, so cortisol is stimulated instead to provide the brain with sugar (glucose) from proteins and fats. It also increases the risk of leaky gut syndrome, lowers SIgA levels, depletes the body of numerous vitamins and minerals, and alters the balance of intestinal bacteria.

Total Score =   /25 (women)

Total Score =   /24 (men)

What's Your Score?

Essentially, the higher your score the more likelihood there is that your level of stress is in excess of what your body can handle without side-effects, which will include digestive disturbances and the risk of food intolerances.

Please be aware that if you have IBS symptoms a lot of the time and feel stressed but your score is low on this questionnaire, then there is the real possibility that your IBS is the cause of your stress rather than the reverse. It is also true that you may feel more stressed because your IBS has diminished your tolerance levels to other stressors in your life.

INTERPRETING YOUR SCORE

0–5

This is where you want your score to be. However, even a score of 4 could mean that adrenal stress maybe affecting how well your digestive system works. Remember, stress sends a message to your brain and then to your body, telling it to prepare to fight or flee and taking energy away from all other functions, including digestion. This is why stress results in decreased blood flow to the digestive system. When this happens symptoms may well ensue, including abdominal bloating, indigestion, burping, wind, constipation or diarrhea – essentially the symptoms associated with Irritable Bowel Syndrome (IBS). All of this is strongly linked with food intolerance.

Suggested Action

Slow down when you eat and chew your food well. Do not eat large meals. Do not eat late at night. Increase your variety of foods to limit the risk of eating too much, too often of a particular food or foods.

6–10

This suggests more long-term stress. The comments for a score of 0–5 apply.

Suggested Action

Slow down when you eat and chew your food well. Make time for your meals. Put your food down in between mouthfuls. Do not work or do anything else while you are eating. Do not eat large meals. Do not eat late at night. Increase your variety of food to limit the risk of eating too much, too often of a particular food or foods. You also need to take measures to reduce the specific markers of excess stress that have been identified in this questionnaire and implement a course of action to address at least one of these every two weeks. Remember, excess stress is potentially a significant cause of food intolerances as well as the digestive symptoms that accompany them.

Follow the Adrenal Support Plan (page 158).

11–15

Please read the comments as for a score of 6–10. This is a high score, and reflects that your level of stress is almost certainly having an impact on your digestive system and risk of food intolerance.

Suggested Action

In addition to following the suggested actions for a score of 6–10, you should test your adrenal hormone levels with the Adrenocortex Stress Profile saliva test (see pages 296–7). Until you get a chance to have the test, start using the Adrenal Support Plan (page 158).

More Than 15

Please read the comments as for a score of 11–15. This is a high score, and reflects that your level of stress is almost certainly having an impact on your digestive system and risk of food intolerance.

Suggested Action

In addition to following the suggested action as for a score of 11–15, you should test your adrenal hormone levels with the Adrenocortex Stress Profile saliva test (see pages 296–7). It is also strongly recommended that you seek some kind of help in order to reduce the excess stress in your life. If you do not get to take the test right away, please start the Adrenal Support Plan at once (see page 158).

Case Study: Food Causes Stress

Jane Grearson, 31, was suffering with a number of health problems. She not only had fatigue, depression, and mood swings but had also put on weight which she swore was NOT related to the amount of food she was eating. Since she was consuming coffee and alcohol every day, these were prime culprits – I told her to stop them for a trial period. I also identified that she was eating an awful lot of wheat, some days at each meal. Therefore, I suggested she have a trial period where she ate alternatives. Jane did these things, suffered withdrawal symptoms after a few days with headaches, but persevered. The next time I saw her, five weeks later, she told me that her mood was significantly better, she had not felt depressed, and her energy levels were much higher. Interestingly, in this case she had not yet lost weight. It took a further four weeks before some of the excess weight began to start coming off.

> **Relevant Tests: Adrenocortex Stress Profile (salivary)**

Summary

Stress is involved in IBS, and IBS itself can cause stress. You may require specific nutritional support to improve your stress tolerance. You can actually measure how your stress hormones are performing with a saliva test, and the appropriate Action Plan can be selected accordingly to reduce your stress and thereby help improve digestive function and reduce the impact and future risk of food intolerance symptoms.

11

Leaky Gut Syndrome

This chapter explains what leaky gut syndrome is, what it does to you, how food intolerances and other things cause it and how it can be measured. This chapter also examines the relationship between a leaky gut and your liver. How to combat the syndrome is explored briefly here and in more detail in Part 3.

Your Intestinal Lining

The intestinal lining, or 'inside skin', can unglamorously be described as a tube approximately 25 foot long, running through the body from the mouth to the anus. It is not exactly a pleasant subject for casual conversation, but this should not detract from its critical importance to your overall health.

Normally, your intestinal lining permits the absorption of nutrients and prevents larger, potentially toxic molecules from getting through. This makes it a selective, semi-permeable barrier. It is only as thick as your eyelid. It is your intestines that ultimately meet the world in the raw, so to speak, and therefore they have developed highly specialized means by which to permit absorption and protect the rest of your body. In fact, as much as 70 percent of your immune cells are located in and along your intestinal lining, to deal with the potential threat that this route presents.

The three main functions of your intestinal lining:

1) selective absorption or transport of nutrients
2) protection against larger, potentially toxic and antigenic molecules from getting into your bloodstream
3) immune protection, which mainly means the secretion of secretory immunoglobulin A (SIgA), which binds to bacteria and other antigens, preventing them from binding to your intestinal lining and thereby enabling them to be eliminated.

The health of your intestinal lining is vital to the health of the rest of your body. If something goes wrong with any of the above three functions, you could end up with increased intestinal permeability, which is commonly known as leaky gut syndrome. On occasions, there could also be decreased permeability, or malabsorption, which may prevent nutrients from being absorbed while, somewhat ironically, still permitting large molecules through, as might be found in celiac disease (gluten allergy).

Somewhat remarkably, any damage to the intestinal lining can be repaired in a matter of about four to five days, whereas injury to your external skin area usually takes about four weeks. It is precisely because of this rapid turnover of cells that your intestinal lining is so vulnerable to the consequences of any interruption to its functions.

What Does Leaky Gut Syndrome Do to Me?

There are a host of problems that can occur if your intestinal lining is more permeable than it should be, allowing molecules to get through when they shouldn't. The absorption of antigenic (allergy or intolerance-provoking) molecules along with unwanted bacteria or yeast from the intestines to other parts of the body can cause problems in every system of the body, from fatigue and brain fog to arthritis and skin conditions. Additionally, leaky gut syndrome has been found alongside a number of other health conditions, as shown in the table below, including rheumatoid arthritis, ankylosing spondylitis, Inflammatory Bowel Syndrome (IBD), eczema, and asthma.

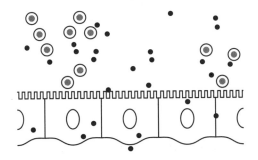

Healthy mucosa allows nutrients to pass the barrier while blocking the entry of toxins.

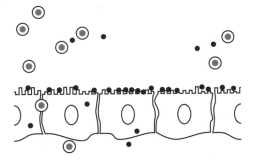

With leaky gut, the barrier is dysfunctional, blocking nutrients at the damaged villi while permitting toxins to enter the bloodstream.

Phase I

Chemical Reactions
Oxidation

Phase II

Chemical Reactions
Sulfation

Reduction

Hydrolysis

Dehalogenation

Glucuronidation

Glutathione Conjugation

Acetylation

Amino Acid Conjugation

Methylation

Nutrients used as enzymes & co-factors

Vitamin B2

Vitamin B3

Vitamin B6

Folic Acid

Vitamin B12

Glutathione

Branched Chain Amino Acids

Flavonoids

Phospholipids

Nutrients used as enzymes & co-factors

Sulfur

Glutathione

Glycine

Taurine

Glutamine

Ornithine

Arginine

* Intermediary Metabolites require sufficient antioxidants of many different types to become quenched successfully.

Leaky Gut and Auto-immune Diseases

Auto-immune diseases are almost always associated with leaky gut syndrome, and reversing auto-immune disease depends in large part on healing the lining of the gastro-intestinal tract. An auto-immune disease is defined as one in which the immune system makes antibodies against its own tissues. Doctors are increasingly recognizing the importance of the gastro-intestinal tract in the development of these conditions.

LEAKY GUT SYNDROME AND CHRONIC FATIGUE

In the same way that auto-immune conditions are associated with leaky gut syndrome, which may also be caused or perpetuated by the presence of food intolerances, so can chronic fatigue (also referred to as Chronic Fatigue Syndrome or ME – myalgic encephalitis). The leaky gut can cause antigens (substances to which the body can create antibodies) to get into your general circulation, and these can get into various tissues and trigger an inflammatory reaction whenever you eat the culprit food. If this inflammation occurs in a joint, auto-immune arthritis (rheumatoid arthritis) develops. If it occurs in the brain, ME (Chronic Fatigue Syndrome) may be the result. Practically any organ or body tissue can become affected by food intolerances that were either involved in creating the leaky gut or were created by the leaky gut itself. Symptoms, especially those seen in conditions such as chronic fatigue syndrome, can be multiple and severely debilitating.

Once you have a better understanding of what happens in leaky gut syndrome, you will be able to see why healing the intestinal lining by eliminating culprit foods and using safe, natural remedies should help not only your immediate issues but also the underlying issues that affect every other aspect of your health.

Conditions Associated with Leaky Gut Syndrome (LGS)

Acute gastroenteritis	Celiac disease
Alcoholism	Crohn's disease
Ankylosing spondylitis	Cystic fibrosis
Alopecia areata	Diabetes (type I)
Arthritis	Eczema
Asthma	Endotoxemia
Burn injury	Fibromyalgia
Chronic fatigue syndrome (CFS)	Food intolerance/allergy

Lupus (SLE)

Multiple sclerosis

NSAID use

Pancreatic dysfunction

Polymyalgia rheumatica

Raynaud's disease

Rheumatoid arthritis

Schizophrenia

Sjögren's syndrome

Surgery

Thyroiditis

Trauma

Ulcerative colitis

Urticaria (hives)

Vasculitis

Vitiligo

Food Intolerances and Leaky Gut Syndrome

Food intolerance is intimately related to leaky gut syndrome, but it is not the only cause. On the one hand, inappropriate and inflammatory immune reactions in the intestines, as triggered by an intolerance reaction to a food, cause an increase in intestinal permeability. This permits large antigenic molecules across the barrier, allowing them to interact with the immune system, creating antibodies, immune complexes and a systemic immune response – and invariably resulting in symptoms. In fact, research shows that those with food intolerances have an increased intestinal permeability compared with controls. In another study investigating children, indications of leaky gut were significantly higher in those with food intolerances.

This means that when you eat foods to which you have an intolerance, you cause leaky gut, to one degree or another. If this happens, not only do food molecules pass through your intestinal lining to cause a problem elsewhere, but there's an increased risk of unwanted bacteria and yeasts, and their toxins, getting through too.

Many of the systemic (throughout-the-body) effects of food intolerances are possible only when your intestinal permeability is compromised. Hence the emphasis on supporting your 'inside skin' if you have a food intolerance.

Case Study: Bloated Leaky Gut

Grace McDonald, 51, complained of excess body fat and almost permanent abdominal bloating. Her diet was pretty good on the whole but there were daily departures consisting mainly of poor snack foods such as doughnuts, cheese, chips, chocolate, and too much coffee.

The degree of bloating suggested the need to rule out a leaky gut, and testing did indeed show that Grace had a leaky gut. I recommended that she avoid the convenience snack foods and replace them with healthier alternatives such as fruit and hummus on wheat-free crackers, and that she avoid all coffee, alcohol, and wheat. Her motivation was high due to her severe bloating.

Grace reported back after a few weeks that her bloating had subsided by about 50 percent and that she had lost nearly 7lb without even trying. She told me that she thought a lot of this was water weight since she had passed a lot of fluids in that short time. In the weeks that followed, Grace reported a complete absence of her bloating. Certainly, water retention is a common symptom associated with food intolerance and leaky gut.

Causes of Leaky Gut Syndrome

The following list is not definitive, but includes the major known causes of increased intestinal permeability.

Eating Foods to Which You Have an Intolerance

In medical terms, this is also known as allergic gastroenteropathy and/or allergic eosinophilic gastroenteropathy. However, altered intestinal permeability can occur long before these states exist. When food intolerances exist, leaky gut syndrome usually follows.

Alcohol

The more alcohol you drink, the greater the degree of intestinal permeability. Part of the reason for this is that alcohol creates a deficiency in N-Acetyl-Glucosamine (NAG), a building-block for the epithelial cells in the intestine. In tests done on alcoholics, markers of intestinal permeability returned to normal after 15 days' abstinence.

Antibiotics

First, antibiotic therapy can inhibit the friendly bacteria that play a key role in maintaining the intestinal lining. Antibiotics also often lead to an overgrowth of unfriendly, competing opportunistic micro-organisms. Antibiotics not only inhibit protective species of bacteria, they may also increase the adherence of yeast to the intestinal wall, as shown in animal research. Altered intestinal ecology and bacterial overgrowth are conducive to the passage, or translocation, of bacteria and yeast into your general circulation. Antibiotics are a cause of this translocation, which is associated with leaky gut syndrome.

Non-steroidal Anti-inflammatory Drugs (NSAIDs)

NSAIDs such as ibuprofen, aspirin and so on all cause a leakiness of the intestinal lining. There are at least three mechanisms by which this occurs:
1. they create a deficiency of N-Acetyl-Glucosamine (NAG)
2. they interrupt the secretion of protective substances called prostaglandins

3. they bind to and prevent the function of the most abundant protective phospho-
   lipid that lines the intestinal lining (it's called dipalmitoylphosphatodylcholine, or
   DPPC). This allows stomach acid to come into contact with the mucosal epithelial (inner skin) cells.

Another potential cause is that NSAIDs disable cellular energy-production, leading
to cell death and a diminished capacity on the part of the cells to heal themselves.
These effects on the intestinal lining appear to the same whether these drugs are
taken orally, intravenously or rectally.

Secretory IgA (SIgA) Insufficiency

This is the most commonly-diagnosed immune deficiency (affecting about 1 in 400
people), and can be caused by excessive stress or exercise. Chronic stress lowers
SIgA – the emotional state of frustration is of particular relevance here. Feelings of
frustration tend to linger for longer than those of anger, and the chronic nature of
frustration is associated with low SIgA. Other challenges to SIgA include food intolerance and bacterial and yeast overgrowth. People with food intolerances have
been found to have too low a level of serum IgA (that is, IgA in the bloodstream).

Corticosteroids

Prednisone, cortisone, and other steroid medications inhibit protein turnover and
suppress immunity, having a negative impact on SIgA levels (since SIgA is an
immune protein) and on the rate at which the intestinal lining heals itself.

Eating Too Much of the Same Foods/Eating Them Too Often

The shocking fact is that as much as 80 percent of the typical diet is
comprised of only 8–10 foods. This does not bode well for our intestinal health,
nor does it say much for achieving a diverse source of nourishment.

Sugar

Refined sugar is an anti-nutrient and feeds unwanted micro-organisms which can have a deleterious effect on intestinal health. Remember that one of the functions of the intestinal tract is an immunological one, and since sugar can weaken immunity for a number of hours after it has been consumed, it can weaken intestinal protection.

Amino Acid Deficiency

Since amino acids are required to nourish the intestinal lining – indeed, as much as 50 percent of the amino acids we consume may feed the intestines directly – a lack of one or more of these building-blocks can contribute to a leaky gut. L-glutamine and N-acetyl-glucosamine (NAG) are the most important, but a variety of others play a role, too, including arginine, taurine and the branched-chain amino acids (leucine, isoleucine, valine).

Zinc and/or Vitamin A Deficiency

Zinc is vital for all growth and healing in the body, and vitamin A is needed for all epithelial growth and repair. These two nutrients are commonly low in the UK diet. Given that vitamin A is fat-soluble, and that most of us eat fewer fatty foods (e.g. liver, full-fat milk) than our forebears did, we may have lower levels of this vitamin than in previous generations. To make things worse, zinc is required to release vitamin A from your liver – so if you're not getting enough of both, you could be compromising your intestinal health.

Digestive Tract Infections

Unwanted, unfriendly bacteria such as *Enterobacter cloacae*, *Klebsiella pneumoniae*, *Citrobacter freundii*, *Proteus* species, *Pseudomonas aeruginosa*, as well as the more famous yet less common *Salmonella* and *E. coli,* can all disrupt normal intestinal ecology and alter intestinal permeability.

Parasites such as *Dientamoeba fragilis*, *Blastocystis hominis*, *Shigella*, and *Histolytica* are also commonly identified in people with leaky gut syndrome.

Yeasts including *Candida albicans* and *Geotrichum* species are also commonly involved in creating and perpetuating a leaky gut.

Stress

This can be caused by a variety of things including endurance or intense prolonged exercise, severe psychological or emotional trauma, or even strong infections. All of these can lead to a leaky gut.

There is an intimate relationship between stress and SIgA, in that stress lowers our intestinal defences, making us more prone to inflammatory reactions after eating and to poor healing on the part of the intestines. Stress also tends to close down the workings of the digestive system as the body diverts blood to the large muscles, in readiness for fight or flight. If this happens often enough, it can lead to a reduced output of hydrochloric acid and pancreatic enzymes, let alone blood flow to the digestive system, which is much needed to digest a meal. (It is for this reason that people are advised to wait an hour or two after they've eaten before swimming: cramps can result because blood flow is occupied with the workings of the digestive system.)

Poor Digestion

This involves one or more of the following:

- underproduction of hydrochloric acid in the stomach (hypochlorhydria)
- underproduction of pancreatic enzymes
- underproduction of bile acids (sluggish gallbladder or liver problems)
- rapid transit of food through the intestine (e.g. diarrhea)

- insufficient chewing or too rapid swallowing of foods.

A lack of digestive juices leads to two main problems related to leaky gut:

1. If you do not digest a food properly, it presents itself as a foreigner that needs to be dealt with by the intestinal immune system. If this happens often enough, it can result in inflammatory reactions within the intestines, leading to increased intestinal permeability and long-term food intolerances.

2. If you lack stomach acid, you lose your front-line sterilizing agent, thereby permitting unwelcome bacteria or yeast to survive and potentially set up home in your intestines.

Inflammatory Bowel Diseases

Crohn's disease, ulcerative colitis, and celiac disease are all conditions in which either increased or decreased intestinal permeability can occur. Since inflammation is a known cause of leaky gut syndrome, it should be no surprise that such conditions can co-exist with leaky gut. There is research that confirms the link with Crohn's disease, and furthermore, those patients with Crohn's in remission whose intestines were leaky were shown to be more likely to suffer a relapse within a year.

Some research has focused on family members of those suffering with Crohn's, and some has shown that there is a positive link with leaky gut (i.e. first-degree relatives of those with Crohn's do have increased intestinal permeability). Other research, however, has not found a link.

Crohn's and colitis are both challenging conditions. However, no matter what medical treatment you are receiving for them, it would be sensible to rule out the presence of food intolerances by measuring your intestinal permeability.

LESS COMMON CAUSES OF LEAKY GUT SYNDROME

Bioflavonoid Insufficiencies

When an antigen, such as a food protein, is exposed to a mast cell, it releases inflammatory substances that include histamine and leukotrienes. The generic term for these chemical messengers is cytokines. These cytokines can promote inflammation in the intestine which can contribute to increased intestinal permeability. Bioflavonoids such as quercetin and luteolin help to temper the release of these inflammatory substances; if there is a lack of these bioflavonoids, the mast cells can be unstable and more prone to release histamine and leukotrienes. This is why some formulae used to treat the intestinal lining contain quercetin.

Famine/Starvation/IV Drip-feeding

Since the intestinal lining is nourished by a local food supply, when this is taken away the normal healing process of the intestinal wall is immediately affected. Of course, there is usually significant stress associated with these processes as well.

Premature Birth

Premature babies are more prone to food intolerances and atopic diseases.

Too Early an Exposure to Whole Foods

While the intestinal lining is developing, if foods are fed to babies before they can properly digest them (before the age of four to six months), this can readily contribute to an aggravated intestinal lining. It is particularly important to help babies get off to a good start in life.

Radiation Therapy to the Abdomen, Uterus or Colon

This cancer treatment has a direct impact on the healing of the intestinal lining, which normally renews itself completely in a matter of days.

Spicy Foods

In some individuals, eating too many chillies can contribute to inflammation of the intestinal lining, which in turn leads to increased intestinal permeability. However, and interestingly, there are also components of chillies, called capsaicins, that have an anti-inflammatory role in the body.

Questionnaire: Have I Got Leaky Gut Syndrome?

Although many of the symptoms associated with food intolerance are identical to those of leaky gut syndrome, the symptoms can be distinguished by looking at the typical causes, as listed on pages 101–9, and those conditions described in the Table on pages 100–1.

SCORING

Score 1 point for each of the questions in Part 1, and 4 points for each of the conditions listed in Part 2.

Please note that conditions for which tests are required (e.g. SIgA and nutrient levels) have been omitted from the questionnaire.

Part 1 (1 Point Each)

Do you (or have you recently) on a regular basis ...

1. Eaten foods to which you have an intolerance?
2. Drunk alcohol on more than 4 nights a week?
3. Taken antibiotics more than twice in a year?
4. Taken steroid medications (e.g. cortisone) for more than one week a year?
5. Taken NSAIDs (aspirin, ibuprofen, etc.) for more than two weeks in a year?

6. Eaten the same foods every day, with a total of fewer than 15 foods comprising the bulk of your diet in any given week?

7. Eaten sugar every day?

8. Had digestive problems such as wind, bloating, discomfort, pain, irregular bowel movements (diarrhea/constipation), reflux, indigestion?

9. Felt that you are anxious or stressed a lot of the time?

10. Gone on extended fasts or starvation diets?

11. Been on an IV drip for whatever reason?

12. Undergone radiation therapy?

13. Undergone surgery?

14. Eaten lots of spicy food?

Also:

15. Were you born premature?

Total Part 1 = /15

Part 2 (4 points each)

Do you suffer from …

1. Colitis or Crohn's disease?

2. Acute gastroenteritis?

3. Alcoholism?

4. Ankylosing spondylitis?

5. Alopecia areata?

6. Arthritis?

7. Asthma?

8. Burn injuries?

9. Chronic fatigue syndrome (CFS)?

10. Celiac disease?

11. Crohn's disease?

12. Cystic fibrosis?

13. Diabetes (type I)?

14. Eczema?

15. Endotoxaemia?

16. Fibromyalgia?

17. Lupus (SLE)?

18. Multiple sclerosis?

19. Pancreatic dysfunction?

20. Polymyalgia rheumatica?

21. Raynaud's disease?

22. Rheumatoid arthritis?

23. Schizophrenia?

24. Sjögren's syndrome?

25. Thyroiditis?

26. Trauma?

27. Ulcerative colitis?

28. Urticaria (hives)?

29. Vasculitis?

30. Vitiligo?

Total Part 2 =

Grand Total =

INTERPRETING YOUR SCORE

The questionnaire does not have a practical maximum total, since it is unlikely that you would have more than a handful of the conditions in Part 2, although Part 1 has a total of 15.

Since the results of a test for intestinal permeability do not give you any indication of what the cause is, taking it is not vital to making a diagnosis of a leaky gut. Therefore, testing for intestinal permeability is only required if you have only a few digestive symptoms (see Food Intolerance Questionnaire, page 6) or if indicated by the results of this questionnaire.

If You Scored Between 1 and 5

If this score derives solely from Part 1, then it is possible you have Leaky Gut Syndrome. Your symptoms should improve by following the Action Plans detailed in this book. If you scored 4 points in Part 2, then it is worth taking the intestinal permeability test. If the results of this test are positive, then add the Gut Lining Plan (pages 158–9) to your existing Action Plan.

If You Scored Between 6 and 9

If this score derives solely from Part 1, then the indications are that you have some degree of leaky gut. Follow the Gut Lining Plan (see pages 158–9) in addition to your existing Action Plan.

If you scored 4 or more points in Part 2, then it is recommend you take the intestinal permeability test in order to get a better idea of the degree of the problem.

If You Scored 10 or Above

It is recommend you take the intestinal permeability test to get a better idea of the degree of the problem. After you have done the test, commence the Gut Lining Plan (see pages 158–9) alongside your existing Action Plan.

How Does Testing for Leaky Gut Syndrome Work?

Measuring the degree of leaky gut involves a urine test. While there are a number of different tests, they all involve swallowing a liquid which contains molecules that have specific absorption characteristics but are not metabolized by the body. The different molecules used for this purpose include: Cr-51-labeled EDTA, mannitol and lactulose, rhamnose, and varying molecule weights and sizes of polyethyleneglycol (PEG).

After fasting overnight, you provide a first morning urine sample which acts as a pre-test specimen. You then drink the solution. Urine is collected over the next six hours and a sample is taken from this. An analysis determines whether you have too many or too few of these molecules, and portrays the results in numerical and graph form.

Both the PEG test and the lactulose and mannitol test provide clinically useful data on the degree of leakiness of your intestinal lining, but they do not tell you the source of the problem. For this reason it is not a front-line test for everyone with food intolerances or digestive problems. However, it is a good test to take if you are not suffering digestive problems but are experiencing a high degree of psychological symptoms. More information on how to access this Intestinal Permeability test is provided in Appendix III.

What Can I Do to Avoid a Leaky Gut?

The simplest thing is to avoid all of the causes outlined above (pages 101–9). Of course, this may be easier said than done. If you are reading this book, you may well have an inkling that there may be a food or two to which you have an intolerance. The information and Action Plans provided in this book should help reduce the risk of leaky gut and/or solve the problem.

How Can I Heal My Leaky Gut?

While eliminating the offending foods, drinks and drugs (e.g. alcohol or NSAIDs) is key, the Gut Lining Plan (see pages 158–9) will also greatly increase your speed of recovery. There are very few instances in which this Plan has not been successful. However, there are two additional considerations here. First, there may well be an underlying cause that is not simply your intolerance to foods. There may be an imbalance in your stress hormones cortisol and DHEA, or there may be an imbalance in your intestinal bacteria levels (intestinal dysbiosis). I would encourage you to complete the questionnaires in earlier chapters, if you have not done so already, to help you identify potential contributory or causative factors.

WHAT CAN HELP THE HEALING PROCESS?

There are a number of nutrients, herbs and so on that nourish the intestinal lining, and others that calm inflammation. Some perform both functions. Here is a list of the most commonly used nutrients and herbs, with a brief description of each one's specific role.

Glutamine – The number-one fuel for the enterocytes (cells of the intestinal lining). The intestinal tract is the principal user of glutamine in the body, but this amino acid has a number of other roles in the body as well. Estimates (in animals) are that 40 percent of the glutamine ingested is used by the intestinal lining. Cells in the large intestine also use glutamine, although short-chain fatty acids (see below) are the main fuel source in the colon. Exercise, illness, injury or infection use up glutamine. As much as 15 gm of glutamine a day has been recommended for healing a leaky gut.

NAG (N-Acetyl-Glucosamine) – Glutamine is also the precursor molecule for glucosamine production in the body. Glucosamine is essential for making mucin, the protective layer in the intestinal wall. Therefore, NAG is an important adjunctive nutrient in supporting the intestinal lining.

Butyric Acid – This is a naturally-occurring short-chain fatty acid found in butter but also made within your intestine. It has a number of functions, primarily limited to the intestine and liver. It is the most important and abundant short-chain fatty acid (SCFA) feeding the cells in the colon. Butyric acid influences the adherence of friendly bacteria in your colon and is vital for maintaining a strong immunity within the bowel. Butyrate, along with other SCFAs, are mainly derived from the fermentation of soluble fiber by colonic bacteria. Oat bran, which contains soluble fiber, increases the level of butyric acid, but wheat brain does not. Other fibers higher in soluble fiber are more effective at increasing butyric acid than oat bran (see below).

Fiber – The roles of fiber (such as cellulose or flax/linseed powder) include the sweeping away of toxins as well as providing the source material from which colonic bacteria make SCFAs to nourish the cells of the colon wall. Fiber also helps to lower the pH of the intestines, thus making it more acidic, which encourages the growth of friendly bacteria and suppresses the growth of unwelcome bacteria such as *Clostridium difficile*.

Lactobacillus bacteria – These lactic acid-forming bacteria lower the intestinal pH and also compete for the nutrients on which potentially unwanted bacteria could feed; they also compete for binding sites on the intestinal wall. In addition, they help to support the production of SIgA. *Lactobacillus casei* GG, in particular, significantly helps the SIgA response in children with Crohn's disease or juvenile chronic arthritis. This improved SIgA response is also likely to help normalize intestinal permeability.

Saccharomyces boulardii – This is a beneficial yeast similar (but not identical) to baker's yeast (*Saccharomyces cerevisiae*), although it is worth pointing out that a typical stool analysis may not be able to distinguish between the two. *S. boulardii* is one of the most effective means known to improve SIgA levels, and thereby help support and protect the intestinal lining. Since it also prevents unwanted bacteria from binding to the intestinal wall and also helps to oust other yeasts, it is a very useful supplement for leaky gut.

Fish oil – This has an anti-inflammatory effect in the intestine by decreasing the production of many inflammatory substances (including leukotrienes) and by increasing the anti-inflammatory prostaglandins derived from the omega 3 fatty acid family, PGE3. Be sure to choose a product made by a company which takes great care in processing and filtering unwanted toxins such as heavy metals and PCBs. The highest-quality products are recommended in the Action Plans in Part 3.

Blackcurrant seed oil, Borage oil or Evening Primrose oil – These omega 6 oils increase the production of the anti-inflammatory prostaglandin family, PGE1.

Gamma oryzanol (from rice) – This nutrient has been found to increase the growth of tissue within the body, including the intestinal lining.

Slippery elm – A traditional and long-used remedy for soothing the stomach.

Quercetin and rutin – Quercetin is perhaps the best-known flavonoid used to help stabilize mast cells to prevent their emission of cytokines (a process called degranulation). Rutin has particular affinity for capillaries, helping to strengthen them.

Aloe vera – A well-known plant, the extracts of which can help with external wounds as well as internal ones such as those along the intestinal lining.

DG-Licorice – This is licorice with the glycyrrhizic acid removed. DG-Licorice has well-documented anti-inflammatory effects in the stomach.

MSM (methylsulfonylmethane) – This contains a bio-available form of sulphur, an element that is present in all living organisms. MSM supports the connective tissue and has been shown to be of benefit in conditions where inflammation, unfriendly microbes and allergens are involved in adverse reactions. It also enhances mucosal membranes.

Ginger root – A traditional anti-inflammatory that also helps reduce nausea (antiemetic).

Phosphatidyl choline – This is one of the body's essential phospholipids (phosphorous combined with fat) that make up the membrane of every cell in the body, including those of the intestine. Therefore, Phos Choline is also a useful nutrient for intestinal lining support. Its main function is as a fat emulsifier and it protects the liver.

Perm A Vite

This is a powder containing a number of the important intestinal-healing nutrients. It was formulated by Dr Leo Galland, a pioneer of Functional medicine in the US. This product consistently reduces intestinal discomfort and almost always produces an improvement in symptoms, as demonstrated by repeat intestinal permeability tests.

The Gut Lining Plan in Part 3 provides you with specific remedies that have proven successful time and again in normalizing intestinal permeability, whether there is leaky gut or malabsorption at the heart of the problem.

Your Liver and Leaky Gut Syndrome

The last topic to discuss in this chapter is the relationship that leaky gut has with your liver. The liver is a multi-functional organ with already enough to do, without the challenge of yet more toxins from your intestine.

In 1989 alone, more than one billion pounds of chemicals were released into the ground, threatening the soil and wildlife and the underground water tables. Over 188 million pounds of chemicals were discharged into lakes and rivers. More than 2.4 billion pounds of chemical emissions were pumped into the air we breathe. A grand total of 5,705,670,380 pounds of chemical pollutants were released into the environment we eat, breathe and live in, all in just one year.

To compromise our bodies' ability handle toxins even further, our food supply has become ever-more refined, processed and devoid of nutritional value. More and more artificial additives, colorings, flavorings and preservatives are being added to our food.

Combine all this with the huge number of digestive complaints suffered by the population (digestive problems are the most common reason people visit their doctor), and the burden on the liver is not insignificant. Food intolerances certainly provide a major source of additional toxin burden for the liver.

Your intestines perform a major role in detoxification, being responsible for up to 50 percent of detoxification in the human body. Environmental and/or intestinal toxins have the potential to diminish optimal health. In good working order, your liver filters out and transforms toxic substances into harmless ones that can be excreted via the bowels or in urine.

When faced with the additional burden of increased intestinal permeability, the liver may fail to perform at a level which promotes good health. In fact, since many of the symptoms affect other parts of the body, rather than just your digestive system, we can know for certain that the immune complex or toxic protein molecules that have escaped from the intestine must also have passed through the liver.

The liver requires a wide array of nutrients to perform its various phases of detoxification, as shown in the diagram below.

LIVER DETOXIFICATION PATHWAYS

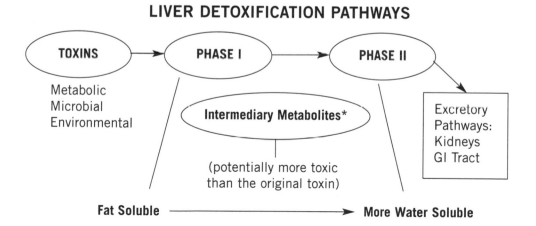

When liver detoxification is not working as it should, it can readily contribute to a host of other conditions not dissimilar to those associated with leaky gut. Just as food intolerance is linked with other conditions in the body such as leaky gut, so too is poor liver detoxification. Chronic Fatigue Syndrome, an increased sensitivity to chemicals, fibromyalgia, arthritis, eczema, headaches, and migraines are particularly associated with poor liver detoxification. However, another cause of poor liver detoxification can be an infection, the ingestion of a poison, or drug misuse. In these instances, specific liver support is recommended as a front-line therapy.

Often, this type of imbalance is also reflected by or associated with a number of digestive symptoms such as poor digestion of fats, nausea, discomfort in the upper abdomen after eating, light, yellow or clay-colored stools, bad breath, and a coated tongue.

CAN I TEST MY LIVER DETOX PROCESSES?

Yes, you can, but not with the standard medical liver function test, which is not precise enough to distinguish which part of the process (divided into Phase I and Phase II) is at the heart of the problem. The better test to take involves a challenge with caffeine, aspirin, and paracetamol, taken separately and then measured in urine or saliva collected afterwards to detect how well your liver has handled these specific agents, which are known to be detoxified along specific pathways. The result gives information on how well these pathways are working. This provides you, and your doctor, with key information about which Phase to support. This is vitally important as you might otherwise exacerbate your symptoms by taking remedies that support a Phase that is already over-working. This is particularly true when Phase I is working faster than Phase II.

In light of this knowledge, the Liver Support Plan (see pages 159–61) contains some general liver-support agents that do not over-stimulate Phase I.

WHEN SHOULD I CONSIDER LIVER SUPPORT?

On the face of it, given the horrific figures describing the volume of toxins 'we' dump on our planet every year, we all could do with some additional liver support. However, if you have conditions such as food intolerance, intestinal dysbiosis, excess yeast or leaky gut, these should be addressed first. You may not get anywhere if you focus on your liver first while these other conditions exist.

I have found that my patients benefit from some liver support at the beginning of their treatment, so you may wish to follow the Liver Support Plan alongside your existing Action Plan.

Summary

You have now learned more about Leaky Gut Syndrome, its causes and the conditions associated with it. You also know now that your liver is the first organ to bear the brunt of any imbalance in intestinal permeability. Your intestinal lining is a gateway through which the most unpleasant immune complexes, toxins, peptides and so on can travel and provoke negative reactions anywhere in your body, potentially leading to auto-immune conditions or chronic fatigue.

Your food intolerances can cause a leaky gut and vice versa, which can create a vicious cycle. If you have food intolerances and digestive problems, then you would certainly do well to nourish your intestinal lining with specific remedies that can reduce inflammation and hasten healing (see the Gut Lining Plan, pages 158–9).

Your liver may well need additional support if you have a leaky gut, but the priorities are to heal the intestinal lining, resolve digestive imbalances and deal with the food intolerances. The longer you have had a leaky gut and digestive problems, the more likely you are to need some liver support (see Liver Support Plan, pages 159–61). More about this can be found in Part 3 (beginning on page 135).

12

The Weight Connection

Can I Really Lose Weight by Avoiding the Foods to Which I Am Intolerant?

The only answer I can offer with any degree of certainty is 'maybe' or 'it depends'. Whilst I have witnessed with my own eyes many clients who have lost weight successfully by avoiding all wheat products, for example, please don't believe all of the claims made for the weight-loss effect of avoiding culprit foods. Everyone is different and what may influence weight loss in some people does not in others.

I cannot guarantee that you will lose weight by excluding the culprit foods causing your intolerance and other symptoms. However, it is true that, for some people, weight loss has undoubtedly been a pleasant side-effect of excluding culprit foods.

In one study of 200 patients using the Food Allergen Cellular Test (FACT) developed by the Individual Wellbeing Diagnostic Laboratory, a number of symptoms were identified as necessary criteria for entering the trial. Twenty-eight (14 percent) of the participants were overweight. All patients avoided the foods which had been identified as causing a positive reaction, for a total of three months. Of these 28 patients, 26 (93 percent) reported weight loss while avoiding the culprit foods. Other studies confirm these observations. Importantly, the authors of the study noted that while weight loss was 'a significant side-effect in many cases', it was not the prime motive for testing or for implementing a change in diet.

This study is discussed in more detail in Chapter 2, where it was also noted that of those participants who had been suffering from Irritable Bowel Syndrome (IBS), 93 percent reported an improvement in their symptoms.

How Is Body Fat Linked with Food Intolerance?

You have learned that there are a host of possible conditions linked with food intolerance, each one of which could be connected in some way with overweight (and sometimes underweight). The more of these conditions you have, the more complex the relationship between weight and food intolerance.

Here are the possible connections:

1. Food addiction
2. Binge-eating
3. Lowered metabolic rate
4. Excess toxicity

Let's take a look in more detail at each of these.

Addiction

Addiction is described as a state involving withdrawal symptoms after contact with a particular substance (these symptoms can be experienced anywhere between a few hours and up to three days afterwards). Just as you can have an addiction to narcotics, tobacco, coffee, or alcohol, you can have an addiction to a chemical or food.

That you could actually be *addicted* to a food you are intolerant to is one of the strangest and most fascinating aspects of food intolerance, and explains a number of things.

First, it helps explain why you may find it difficult, on an emotional level, to accept that a certain, favorite food is causing a problem. It also helps explain why, for some, it is a struggle to eliminate the culprit food(s). You will often crave the food, as it makes you feel good initially even though it is increasing your body's toxicity burden.

This also explains how you can over-eat such foods, and even binge on them. It has to be said that, as with alcohol, it is rarely the foods themselves that are addictive per se, just that there is something in them that reacts with something in you and makes them addictive to you.

Once you accept the addictive aspect of food intolerance, you will be better able to deal with the impact of cutting out your culprit foods. Some of you may be aware that you crave the foods that cause your symptoms, while others may be unwittingly choosing their culprit foods time and again. This is particularly easy to do with wheat and dairy products, since they are so readily available.

The research available indicates that about half of the people with food intolerances will have addictions to those foods.

This is one of the key distinguishing factors of a food intolerance and true food allergy: with a food intolerance, you can feel better initially after eating the food (before feeling worse later on); with an allergy, your initial, immediate reaction will be unpleasant (and in some cases life-threatening).

It is because you get an initial satisfaction and sense of well-being from eating the food that you eat it again. It is therefore difficult to stop eating the food, because this means giving up that good feeling.

As with other addictions, if you avoid the substance to which you are addicted, you will experience withdrawal. In fact, if you get cravings for and experience withdrawal symptoms after eliminating a certain food that you eat regularly, then you will know you are on the right track. It is also true that the cravings will normally disappear in time.

The trouble is that it is all too easy to return to eating the culprit foods after your symptoms improve, especially since there is no control on their availability as there is with drugs. The foods are right there on the shelf.

As you may experience the same type of withdrawal that drug addicts experience, it is important to be aware of what might happen.

HOW DO I GET ADDICTED TO A FOOD?

Remember that you only develop an intolerance to the foods you eat most often. What we are really talking about here is a chemical addiction to something in these foods.

Thanks to the work of researchers such as Candace Pert PhD, author of *The Molecules of Emotion*, we now know more about the intricate workings of the brain. Our body has the ability to make endorphins, which are natural opioids and pain-killers that are released during intense pain and even certain types of exercise. (Endurance or strenuous exercise, for example, causes the release of endorphins – long-distance running encourages the release of more endorphins than other types of cardiovascular exercise, which might explain how people can become addicted to it.)

Endorphins travel to the brain and attach to opiate receptors there, helping to switch off pain and encourage a sense of well-being. You will have heard of morphine, heroin, and other opiates; they bind to these same receptors. These drugs are also very addictive because they inhibit the body's natural ability to produce endorphins, so that when the drugs are stopped the patient or addict suffers tough withdrawal symptoms. In the same way, the foods that trigger the release of opioids in the brain decrease your brain's ability to make more of these chemicals.

Endorphins are comprised of short chains of amino acids called peptides. Proteins are made up of longer chains of amino acids. When foods are digested in the stomach, the proteins in those foods are broken down from these long-chain amino acids into peptides. By some quirk of nature, some of the peptides derived from food are almost identical to our endorphin peptides. The name given to these peptides is exorphins, because they come from *outside* the body. Exorphins can be derived from a variety of foods including wheat, maize, barley, and milk.

One of the questions that arises from this knowledge is why does this affect some people and not others? We don't have all the answers, but we know about some of the variables that play a role. Intestinal permeability (leaky gut) may be a factor, as discussed in Chapter 11, since this could permit more of these peptides through the intestinal lining. The balance of bacteria within your intestine may play a role, too, as discussed in Chapter 6. The levels of stomach acids and digestive enzymes could also be very important, since this could prevent the body from turning the exorphin peptides into benign amino acid chains. This is why digestive enzymes such as Bio 6 Plus comprise a part of the Digestive Support Plan.

Your SIgA levels also provide an important protective layer which peptides cannot easily cross. In fact, many of the factors discussed in this book (Chapters 3–11) surrounding food intolerance could well have implications for how exorphins might be affecting you. In addition, there may be something awry with your detoxification enzymes (located mainly in the intestines and liver) which also play a role in allowing these peptides into your circulation and into your brain.

Case Study: Weight Loss and More ...

Kyle Murray, 57, told me about his long-term health issues and admitted that he knew he ate the wrong foods, but loved them so much. He was nearly 30 lb overweight, was tired most of the time, lacked motivation and had sore knees and his tongue was very coated and too white. He also suffered from frequent (monthly) infections and had asthma, for which he took medication, and a niggling, chronic cough.

So many of these were signs of food intolerance, I told Kyle to avoid his top culprits for a trial period. These turned out to be coffee, alcohol, bread, cheese and milk. In 10 weeks' time Kyle reported back to me, and asked me if I could believe that he had made significant improvements in every single one of his conditions. He told me that whenever he ate cheese his knees hurt and he needed to take his asthma medication more often. His body fat was shrinking day by day and he had gained a new lease of life with much greater motivation than before.

Kyle is a great example of someone who you would never think would ordinarily seek advice from a nutritionist, but he had read about someone like him in a popular magazine. He felt that he had reached the end of the line in his health and was fed up feeling so lousy. His commitment to the program was tested from time to time, but each time he ate or drank the 'culprit' foods or drinks he experienced a worsening of his symptoms, and this reinforced his desire to stick with it.

N.B. Never stop or change the dose of any medication without your doctor's advice.

Binge-eating

This is intimately linked with the biochemical addiction you can have to foods, but there may well be an additional emotional component that starts it all off. When you get upset, you may reach for comfort foods. Some people over-eat in the face of stress or anxiety. Typically, the foods that you eat at these times are high up on the list of Usual Suspects. If you over-eat these foods on a regular basis, it is all the more likely that these are the foods to which you will become addicted, not just biochemically but emotionally as well.

If eating a food too much and too often is the number-one cause of food intolerance, then binge-eating a food time and again is a sure-fire way of developing an intolerance to it. You also run the risk of consuming too many calories and putting on weight, while continuing to crave that food. This could well lead to Leaky Gut Syndrome, which in itself increases the toxicity load within the body. Most of these toxins are stored in fat cells, so this could lead to increased body fat of the kind that resists being used for energy (a process called oxidization).

Lowered Metabolic Rate

Food intolerance can deplete your hormonal system, which can then reduce the body's ability to use fat for energy. This can happen in three ways.

First, whenever you eat a food that triggers a reaction, it stimulates the nervous system and adrenal gland to produce stress hormones. If this only happens now and again, this will not result in any imbalance. However, when this happens regularly and repeatedly it leads to weakness, fatigue and nervousness. The adrenal hormones become depleted and are unable to maintain your metabolic rate effectively. In addition, since all hormones interact with each other, this has a knock-on effect throughout the body, and particularly on the thyroid hormone. In the short term the thyroid hormones can compensate for the sluggish adrenal output, but in time the thyroid gland may also under-produce, leading to thyroid hypo-function. This slows down your metabolic rate – and the slower your metabolism, the more likely you are to put on weight.

Secondly, hormonal glands in the body can be adversely affected by the antibodies that have developed to attack food proteins. Thyroiditis is an example of an auto-immune condition that immune-complexes to food can trigger.

Thirdly, hormones in the body may be disrupted or made less effective by the toxins, cytokines and immune-complexes that result from food intolerances. Insulin function is known to be adversely affected by TNF-a, an inflammatory cytokine that is produced in the intestines as a result of food-intolerance reactions. If insulin cannot do its work, more insulin is made; this leads to a condition called *insulin resistance* (this is the subject of my first book, *The Insulin Factor*). Insulin resistance is strongly associated with weight gain.

However, it is not only insulin that is affected by a food intolerance. This disruption can affect the metabolic function and clearance of all hormones, resulting in hormonal imbalances throughout the body. It can also lead to problems with the body's ability to convert the inactive thyroid hormone to active thyroid hormone.

Toxicity

Toxicity prevents cells from working properly. This also slows down your metabolic rate. Toxicity from food intolerances may well overwhelm the liver's capacity, allowing toxins to enter the bloodstream. This situation typically results in nutrient insufficiency and poor circulation, both of which lead to reduced metabolic activity.

When the body is faced with an excess level of toxins, it will look to store them out of harm's way. This almost always means storing the toxins in fat. In this way, the store of body fat becomes increasingly full of toxins that the body is resistant to breaking down lest it release those toxins back into the circulation.

Excess toxicity can also lead to water retention, a common feature of food intolerance. The body is doing its best to dilute the toxins and inflammation caused by food intolerance. Most people who avoid their culprit foods experience a rapid loss of water weight, usually in the first week of an exclusion diet. This should be distinguished from fat loss, however.

Case Study: Weight Loss and Water Retention

Dina Lacey, 43, really struggled with her weight. She could not understand how she had put on weight and not been able to lose it despite NOT eating too many calories. Upon close examination of her food intake I discovered that she was eating too many of her calories in the form of wheat-based foods. There was also a lot of hidden sugar in these foods and they contained processed fats, which are not healthy at all. When I added up her caloric intake she was not eating more than 2,000 calories a day, and combined with the exercise she did, it did seem strange that she was not losing weight.

However, Dina was a woman for whom the common-sense advice of 'Stop eating these foods for a month and see how you get on' would not wash, so I recommended a food intolerance test. Although these tests do not always reveal *all* the problematic foods, I was very pleased to see that both wheat and sugar appeared on her shortlist of intolerances.

Dina avoided her culprit foods and was more than pleased to discover that she began to lose weight and that her body shape changed, too. Furthermore, she told me that she actually felt better in herself but in a way that was unrelated to her delight at losing weight. We have now actually increased her caloric intake of healthier foods to help support her metabolism and her energy levels.

Summary

Food intolerances can be linked to excess body fat, but not for everyone who is overweight nor for everyone with a food intolerance. The link will be stronger in some than others.

Addressing your food intolerances and other conditions will help you maintain a healthy metabolism, which can lead to weight loss (or weight gain if you are underweight).

There are some very good reasons why a diet that excludes your culprit foods may result in weight loss. These reasons include addiction and compulsive over-eating, interruption of normal hormonal and cellular metabolism, and the body's innate method of dealing with toxicity.

Whether or not you would like to lose weight, you are encouraged to follow the recommendations outlined in the next chapter. That chapter will explain how you should proceed.

Part Three

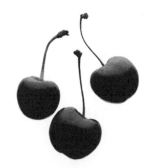

Your Action Plan to Beat Food Intolerance

13

Food Intolerance Action Plan

This chapter puts it all together for you. You will be reminded about how to eliminate culprit foods and how to reintroduce them, how to know what tests to take, and finally what action you can take to support any underlying health issues. Have your questionnaire scores to hand to help you choose the Action Plan that is most appropriate for you.

Food Intolerance Is the Priority

The priority is to do as much as you can to identify and eliminate foods to which you might be intolerant. Once that has been done, you can also identify whether you need to address other conditions linked to food intolerance.

Is There No Cure?

I wish there were a cure for food intolerance. Unfortunately, there is no simple remedy for a condition that is a manifestation of the body's inability to adapt to a number of things, not least eating too much of the same foods too often. By following the recommendations in this book, you will reduce or even eliminate your symptoms.

A Complex Condition

There is no denying that food intolerance is a particularly complex condition given its relationship with many other 'imbalances' described in Part 2. These other problems can be difficult to resolve. Experience with helping many hundreds of clients through this maze has taught me the importance of a clear-cut approach.

Because there are so many variables involved, I have detailed a step-by-step guide. I make no apology for providing you with so much information in this book about the factors that influence food intolerance, because without addressing the related conditions, the efforts of following an elimination diet may be for nothing.

Your Questionnaire Scores

Rest assured that the time you spend completing the questionnaires in this book will be time well spent.

Here is a list of the questionnaires so that you can see at a glance which ones you scored highest on.

Questionnaire	Out of	High Score	My Score
1. Food Intolerance Questionnaire	131	36 or more	
2. Have I got low stomach acid?	15	5 (incl first two) or 7 (excl first two)	

Questionnaire	Out of	High Score	My Score
3. Have I got low digestive enzymes?	12	7 or more	
4. Have I got a yeast overgrowth?		180 (women)	
		140 (men)	
5. Have I got parasites?	25	15 or more	
6. Have I got stress-related digestive problems?	24/25	15 or more	
7. Have I got Leaky Gut Syndrome?		10 or more	

An Overview of Your Action Plan

Although there is quite a lot to food intolerance, there is a simple way forward:

1. Identify food intolerances.

2. Exclude those foods, and reintroduce them later.

3. Support digestive function with the Digestive Support Plans.

4. Identify imbalances in other aspects of your health and take steps to address them while monitoring your progress.

5. Improve other aspects of your health, along with addressing and improving your food intolerance status.

6. Support liver detoxification.

7. Implement the Long-term Action Plan Principles (see pages 147–8) and review your progress.

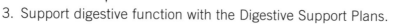

Your First Step

This section provides you with your first step on the road to recovery from food intolerances, and is based on your score in The Food Intolerance Questionnaire. You have already been advised about what to do in Chapter 1, but here is a reminder.

Your Score	Action
Total = 0–15	Exclude the top two foods compared to the Usual Suspects.
Total = 16–25	Exclude the top four foods compared to the Usual Suspects; follow Digestive Support Plan.
Total = 26–35	Exclude top six foods compared to the Usual Suspects, follow Digestive Support Plan.
Total = 36–50	Food Intolerance Lab Test OR Pulse Test; follow Digestive Support Plan and next-most relevant Plan.
Total = 51–70	Food Intolerance Lab Test and next-most important test; follow Digestive Support Plan.
Total = >71	Food Intolerance Lab Test and visit a nutritionist.
Total = > 36	– and your combined score for Sections 2 and 3 is more than double those for Section 1: Intestinal Permeability Test.

Your Next Steps

Your next steps involve your scores to the other questionnaires in the book. Even if you score highly in all the questionnaires, you should follow no more than two plans at once (that is, the two you scored highest on). If in any doubt, follow Digestive Support Plan 1.

Questionnaire
& Your Score   **Action**

The Food Intolerance Questionnaire (high = 51 or more out of 131)

16–25   Elimination/Challenge Diet with Digestive Support Plan 1 for
               at least 1 month

26–35   Elimination/Challenge Diet with Digestive Support Plan 1 for at
               least 2 months. Pulse test or Food Intolerance Test

36–50   Pulse test or Food Intolerance Test, then Exclusion Diet with
               Digestive Support Plan 1 for at least 3 months; reintroduce
               foods after 3 months. Then re-do questionnaire. If score is 15
               or more, do the Intestinal Permeability Test. Follow Gut Lining
               Plan if positive. If negative, do the next most important test
               (if there is one) according to your results on the different
               questionnaires. If positive, follow the relevant Plan. If negative,
               do the next-most important test (if there is one).

51–70   Food Intolerance Test then Exclusion Diet with Digestive
               Support Plan 1 for at least 3 months. Also do next-most
               important test (if there is one). If positive, follow the relevant
               Plan (as well). If negative, do the next most important test
               (if there is one). If that test is positive, then follow the relevant
               Plan. If negative, do the Intestinal Permeability Test. If positive,
               then follow the Gut Lining Plan. If negative, do the next-most
               important test (if there is one). Reintroduce foods after 3
               months. Then re-do questionnaire. If your score is not 15 or

lower then it is recommended to seek the help of a
nutritionist/doctor familiar with this area.

>36   If your total score is 36 or more, and your scores for Section
            Two and Three are greater than double the total of Section One
            then, in addition to the above recommendations, do the
            Intestinal Permeability Test. If positive, then follow the Gut
            Lining Plan. If negative, follow the directions above.

**In addition to the above Action Plan, there are some other important conditions and
imbalances to rule out. Only if you score highly on the relevant questionnaires
should you follow the recommendations made. If you score highly on many questionnaires, then proceed one by one in sequence through the list of questionnaires and
their recommendations as presented below.**

**Questionnaire
& Your Score   Action**

Low Stomach Acid (high = 5 (incl first two) out of 15 or 7 out of 15 (excl first two)
>5–7/15   If you test positive for low stomach acid levels, do the test for
                 H. pylori. If negative, then follow directions as above. If this
                 test is positive, then follow the Anti-*H. pylori* Plan for 6 weeks,
                 together with Digestive Support Plan 1. After 6 weeks follow
                 Digestive Support Plan 2.

Low Digestive Enzymes (high = 7 out 12)
>7/12   Follow Digestive Support Plan 3 for 1 month, then re-do the
                questionnaire. If your score is unchanged or higher than it was

before, then revert back to Digestive Support Plan 1. If your score is less, then continue for 2 more months and then re-do the questionnaire.

Yeast Overgrowth (high = 180 for women, 140 for men)

>180(w)/>140(m) Have the Yeast Culture stool analysis done. If positive for either test, follow the Anti-Yeast Plan in addition to Digestive Support Plan 1 for 3 months, then re-do the questionnaire. Also follow a diet which omits sugar, yeast, alcohol, fruit juices, all soft fruit, white flour products, and mushrooms (see below).

Parasites (high = 15 out of 25)

>15/25   Do the Comprehensive Parasitology Stool Test. If positive, then follow the Anti-Parasitic Plan as well as the Parasite Prevention Plan. Do this for 6 weeks in addition to Digestive Support Plan 1. After two weeks of stopping the Anti-Parasitic Plan, re-do the questionnaire. If your score is still 10 or more, then re-do the Comprehensive Parasitology Test to identify whether or not you have eradicated the parasite(s) identified in the first test. If negative (i.e. no parasites), then proceed with Digestive Support Plan 1 and exclusion of culprit foods, and move on to the next-most important condition if there is one. If positive, then follow the Anti-Parasitic Plan for a further 6 weeks. Do not follow this for more than two courses. After two weeks of stopping the Anti-Parasitic Plan (second time around) re-do the questionnaire. If negative (i.e. no parasites), then proceed with Digestive Support Plan 1. If positive, then seek advice

from a nutritionist/doctor familiar with parasites and food intolerance.

Stress-related Digestive Problems (high = 15 out of 25 for women and 24 for men)

>15(w)/>24(m)   Do the Adrenocortex Stress Profile which measures for cortisol and DHEA. There are many different possible variations of these results, so you are recommended to email me personally so that I can send you the appropriate Remedial Plan for your specific results. Also, you are recommended to make some lifestyle changes as outlined later in this section. If the results are normal, then implement the lifestyle changes, follow the Adrenal Support Plan for 2 months and continue with your exclusion diet and Digestive Support Plan.

Leaky Gut Syndrome (high = 10 or more)

>10   Do the Intestinal Permeability Test. If your gut has altered intestinal permeability, then follow the Gut Lining Support Plan, together with Digestive Support Plan 1 and Exclusion Diet, for 8 weeks. After 8 weeks, re-do the questionnaire. If your score is 10 or more, continue with the same two Plans for a further month. Then re-do the questionnaire. If your score is 9 or less then finish and stop the Gut Lining Support Plan, but re-do the questionnaire in a month's time to ensure that it is still 9 or less. If your score continues to be elevated in spite of following the Plans, then review the other questionnaires to identify if there is another condition which is affecting your intestinal permeability. No matter what, re-do the Intestinal Permeability Test 3 months after having done the first one.

Liver Support

Once you have successfully reduced all your high scores, or if you did not score highly in any in the first instance, you are recommended to embark on a Liver Support Plan. Do this for 3 months, and then re-do the Food Intolerance Questionnaire. If you make no progress and you have done the relevant tests, as above, then make a list of your top ten 'complaints' (e.g. fatigue, muscle pain, abnormal tiredness, etc.) and do the Hepatic Detox Profile. If normal, then you have ruled out that there is an imbalance in this aspect of your health, and it may be worthwhile seeing a nutritionist or doctor to help you make progress. If you have a raised Phase I compared to Phase II then follow Liver Support Plan II, but if your Phase I is lower than Phase II then follow Liver Support Plan III. Do this for 2 months, and then reassess your health by reviewing your top ten complaints and determining whether they have improved.

Anti-yeast Diet

There are many books written on the subject of yeast and *Candida albicans*. The recipes in this book will help anyone who wants to avoid feeding the yeast within their intestines. The other most important foods and drinks to avoid are as follows:

- All alcohol, especially wine and beer
- Juices of all kinds
- Soda pop
- Fruits other than apples and pears
- Refined carbohydrates (such as white rice, white rice flour)
- More than a moderate portion of carbohydrate at any one meal
- Mushrooms

Parasite-prevention Plan

Since parasites are difficult to treat, the adage of an ounce of prevention is worth a pound of cure certainly applies here, since prevention is the best solution. The best line of defense against these opportunistic UFOs is a strong and healthy immune system. Here's a Parasite-prevention Plan that will help you stay parasite-free.

1. Drink filtered, or even boiled-then-cooled water, and always ensure that your food is thoroughly cooked.
2. Eat organic foods, but make sure to wash them thoroughly.
3. Wash your hands with soap before eating. Keep your fingernails short and make sure to wash under the nails.
4. Support your immunity by minimizing stress levels – since stress readily reduces SIgA levels.
5. Cook food at the right temperature to kill parasites (and bacteria). This is 180°C/350°F. Cook meat at a temperature of at least 170°C/325°F. Bake fish at 200°C/400°F for 8–10 minutes per inch of thickness.
6. Beware of or avoid raw foods such as sushi (Japan, China and Korea have a high incidence of infection from raw fish).
7. Sanitize all toilet seats and bowls, particularly those used by children, and always wash your hands thoroughly after changing a diaper.
8. Don't walk barefoot in warm, moist, sandy soil.
9. Don't use tap water to clean contact lenses. Use sterilized lens solutions.
10. Keep toddlers away from puppies and kittens that have not been regularly dewormed, and do not let them kiss animals.

Lifestyle Changes to Reduce Stress

Here are some suggestions that are especially for you if you scored highly in the Have I Got Stress-related Digestive Problems?

1. Stop activities that are not directly helpful to your work, social life or economic goals. Schedule more time for appointments or other tasks. Wake up 15–20 minutes earlier than usual.
2. Create a more relaxed or peaceful environment for work. Organize, get rid of paper and other clutter, add some personal objects such as artwork, toys, etc.
3. Think before you speak – try not to blurt out the first thing that comes to your mind.
4. Plan to spend some time alone daydreaming, talking with friends about non-work activities, browsing in a book store or library.

Long-term Action Plan

Once you have improved your health, following a small number of principles can help you remain well and completely free of food intolerances:

LONG-TERM ACTION PLAN PRINCIPLES

1. Eat a varied diet of whole, non-processed, non-refined foods
2. Try to eat more than 25 different foods a week.
3. Relax before you eat and chew your food thoroughly.
4. Eat small and regular meals, even if this means eating 4 or 5 times a day.
5. Re-do the questionnaires every four to six months to make sure that you are on track.
6. Eat foods in season, where possible, and as many foods as you can that are grown locally, or at least domestically.

7. Get regular exercise, but not intensively more than once a week.

8. Get an hour's daylight every day.

9. Just because you can eat them again, do not over-eat any of the foods to which you have had an intolerance in the past. Eat them on a rotation basis.

10. Avoid stimulants such as nicotine and caffeine, and limit your alcohol intake to 1 glass a day.

14

Elimination and Challenge
or Exclusion Diet?

There are two types of approach recommended to you. First, the Food Elimination/Challenge Diet will be detailed for you. This is to be followed if you are choosing to identify specific foods as intolerant for yourself WITHOUT having done a lab test or pulse test. This is a means of diagnosis. To support your digestive system you should follow Digestive Support Plan 1.

The other approach is one in which you have found out what you are intolerant to and you are going to implement an Exclusion Diet, avoiding those foods without the need to reintroduce them in the short term. You will also review the scores to your questionnaires and decide which Supplement Plan(s) may be of most help to you. Remember, the supplement plans are designed to hasten the process by which you can attain normal, good health.

Either way, it means that you will be changing what you eat and you will need alternatives, and this is what this book is going to help you with.

The Elimination/Challenge Diet

This dietary approach replaces the need for lab or other tests – you are the one who gets to find out what you are intolerant to first, if you did not know already. It is an experiential process. Aim to eliminate the chosen foods for a minimum of two weeks and a maximum of four. If your symptoms are food-related, then most should disappear by the end of the first week, although the antigen-antibody complexes may take a little longer to clear. It is vital that none of the foods on your list is consumed during this time.

WHAT CAN I EXPECT DURING THE ELIMINATION PHASE?

If you have any food intolerances, then you should expect to go through a withdrawal period. Do not mistake a craving for a certain food as an indication that the food is good for you and that you should eat it. You can relieve food cravings by taking a supplement powder called XCravings (see the Anti-Cravings Plan, page 161).

The fewer the number of food intolerances, the easier it is to verify them with this type of approach. If there are multiple food intolerances, it may be very difficult for you to avoid all the culprits, and this may mean that your symptoms do not totally subside. Nonetheless, the process will undoubtedly produce some key information.

CHALLENGE PHASE

Number your culprit foods in ascending order, starting at 1. This is the order in which you are going to reintroduce them to your diet after the two week Elimination Diet. Introduce a food from your list every 4 days, but only eat it once and then avoid it again. Be aware that reintroducing a food you are intolerant to can produce a more severe reaction than before. Therefore, you must keep a detailed record of what foods were reintroduced, when and what symptoms appeared, if any. Here is a suggested layout for your record sheet:

	Date & time reintroduced	Symptoms experienced (date & time)	Avoided for 2 weeks, with 4-day gap between reintroduction
Food 1			
Food 2			
Food 3			
Food 4			
Food 5			
Food 6			

For those of you who have experimented with the Pulse Test (see Appendix I), then this is a good time to implement it.

If you experience a dramatic symptom, you will have the reward of the time and discipline you have put into the process and it should be easier to continue to avoid the food that triggered it. Write down your reaction on the record sheet.

If your existing symptoms do not disappear with this Elimination/Challenge Diet, you may not have avoided all the foods responsible for causing your symptoms, or you may have a number of other conditions co-existing alongside the intolerance(s). Have a look at your questionnaire scores to see which areas are the most likely candidates, and consider following the recommended course of action, be it a lab test or a Supplement Plan.

FOR HOW LONG DO I NEED TO AVOID A FOOD?

Once you know your culprit foods, you should avoid them for between one and nine months. After this time, these foods may be re-introduced carefully. Note any adverse reactions and eat them on a rotation basis thereafter. The longer you avoid these foods, the more likely you are to be successful in overcoming your intolerance. Therefore, it is recommended that you avoid known culprit foods for at least two months before reintroducing them. If, however, you then return to eating large quantities, you may well re-create the same intolerance as before.

A variable that is relevant here is the nature of the other conditions from which you suffer. Do you have Leaky Gut Syndrome? Do you have dysbiosis? Do you have high stress levels? Do you have any of the connected conditions discussed in Part 2? If you have, you need to resolve them at the same time you are avoiding the foods you are intolerant to. It may take between three and nine months to resolve these other issues, and will mean you will be more actively engaged in the process during that time.

HOW LONG WILL IT TAKE FOR MY SYMPTOMS TO DISAPPEAR?

If a food intolerance is the sole cause of a symptom, it can take up to several weeks before the symptom will resolve. This is because the antigen-antibody complexes must be cleared from your system – a process than can take some time. Other symptoms may clear up more quickly (remember how quickly Sally Ann improved her health when she avoided wheat [see pages xvi–xvii]).

WRITE DOWN YOUR MAJOR HEALTH COMPLAINTS

Both approaches take some effort on your part, so it is worth reminding yourself of why you need to do them. To help achieve this, write down a list of your five major complaints (or all of them if you have fewer than this) and put it somewhere you can see it every day. This will serve as a daily motivating factor while you apply yourself to changing your diet. Your efforts really are worth it.

WRITE DOWN YOUR CULPRIT FOODS

It is also imperative that you write down the foods that you are to avoid, whether tested and known or untested possibilities, on a list, and it is best to memorize it, too. Remember to identify alternatives (many of which are provided in this book) so that you can have these to hand and plan to eat these instead.

One of the most practical ways to identify alternatives is to review your existing food intake and then give yourself two alternative meal plans for each meal of the day in which one of your culprit foods appears. This should be possible using the recipes in this book. This means that right away you have a firm idea about what foods you can and will eat.

The next thing to do is to fix a date and start your Elimination/Challenge Diet or Exclusion Diet.

Removing foods you have an intolerance to, such as wheat and dairy products and soy, requires immense attention to detail; even some foods that you might not expect to contain such items can have them as 'hidden' ingredients – check all labels.

15

Your Supplement Plan

Digestive Support Plan 1

This is the mainstay Plan designed to support digestion, reduce inflammation and histamine-release and support the balance of your good bacteria. It is designed to be taken in conjunction with all other Plans except Digestive Support Plans 2 or 3, which are variations on the theme.

Digestive Enzymes

Biotics Research	Bio 6 Plus (pancreatic enzymes)	1 at each meal
P.M.N. (vegetarian formula)	Kristazyme	1 at start of each meal

Well-researched probiotic

Culturelle	*Lactobacillus* GG	1 at breakfast

Anti-inflammatory, anti-histamine, gut-lining support

Allergy Research	GastroCort	2–3 capsules before each meal

(incl. Glutamine, Quercetin, NAG)

Digestive Support Plan 2

Hydrochloric Acid Replacement

Biotics Research	Betaine Plus HP	1 in the middle of each meal (do not take after a meal or without food)

Digestive Enzymes

Biotics Research OR	Bio 6 Plus (pancreatic enzymes)	1–2 at each meal
P.M.N. (vegetarian formula)	Kristazyme	1 at start of each meal

Well-researched probiotic

Culturelle	*Lactobacillus* GG	1 at breakfast

Anti-inflammatory, anti-histamine, gut-lining support

Allergy Research	GastroCort	2–3 capsules before each meal

(incl. Glutamine, Quercetin, NAG)

Digestive Support Plan 3

Digestive Enzymes

Biotics Research	Bio 6 Plus	3 at each meal
OR	(pancreatic enzymes)	
P.M.N. (vegetarian formula)	Kristazyme	1 before, with and after each meal

Well-researched probiotic

Culturelle	*Lactobacillus* GG	1 at breakfast

Anti-inflammatory, anti-histamine, gut-lining support

Allergy Research	GastroCort	2–3 capsules before each meal

(incl. Glutamine, Quercetin, NAG)

N.B. You can also add Betaine Plus HP to this program should you find you need it.

Anti-*H. pylori* Plan

Biotics Research	Bio-HPF	3 capsules in between meals twice daily
Allergy Research	Mastica	3 capsules in between meals twice daily

Anti-Yeast Plan

(Use 1 pot of the Allergy Research product and then 1 pot of the BioCodex product)

| Allergy Research | *Saccharomyces boulardii* | 1 capsule before breakfast & dinner rotate this with: |
| BioCodex | Florastor Lyo *(S. boulardii)* | 2 capsules before breakfast & dinner |

Rotate use of these two products:

| Biotics Research | Caprin (caprylic acid) | build up slowly to 1 at each meal; after 7 days, start building up to 2 at each meal |
| Biotics Research | FC-Cidal (includes Pau D'Arco) | 1 at each meal |

N.B. As a precaution, even though it is indicated for those with a yeast overgrowth, for those of you who have a strong allergy to yeast, please DO NOT take S. boulardii.

Anti-Parasite Plan

(When parasites have been identified in the stool analysis)

Patented anti-parasitic product

| Biotics Research | A.D.P. | 5 at each meal for 7 days, then 3 at each meal and 3 at bedtime for 35 days |

Anti-parasitic plant extract

Allergy Research	Artemisinin	1 capsule at breakfast and dinner (do not take antioxidants at the same time)

Adrenal Support Plan

Ancient French adrenal-stamina tonic

Allergy Research	Stabilium	4 capsules first thing for 2 weeks then 2 capsules first thing for 2 weeks

Herbal support for the adrenals

Allergy Research	3X Ginseng Tea	add hot water to 1 tsp powder in the morning – 1–2 cups daily

Vitamin C – much needed by the adrenal glands

Biotics Research	Bio C Plus (500 mg Vit C)	1 mid-morning & mid-afternoon

Gut Lining Plan

(Chapter 11 describes the nutrients needed for a healthy gut lining. The products containing the most important nutrients are detailed below).

Effective remedy formulated by Dr Leo Galland

Allergy Research	Perm A Vite powder	1 heaped tablespoon

blended in water, taken
30 minutes before meals
twice a day

Probiotic yeast that improves gut lining defences incl. SIgA

Allergy Research	*Saccharomyces boulardii*	1 before at breakfast and dinner (20–30 minutes before food – or in between meals)

Rotate with this:

BioCodex	Florastor Lyo *(S. boulardii)*	2 capsules before break-fast & dinner

(Use 1 pot of Allergy Research product followed by 1 pot of the BioCodex product.)

Important fuel source for cells lining the gut

Biotics Research	Butyric Cal Mag	2 capsules with each meal

N.B. As a precaution, even though it is indicated for those with a yeast overgrowth, for those of you who have a strong allergy to yeast, please DO NOT take S. boulardii.

General Liver Support Plan

Multi-nutrient formula

Allergy Research	Fast & Be Clear Powder	1 tsp in water twice daily for 3 days, then 2 tsp in

water twice daily for 3
days with or away from
food, then 3 tsp in water
twice daily for 3 days,
then 1 scoop twice daily
thereafter

Liver Support Plan – Higher Phase I than II

(When this has been proved by a liver detox test)

Traditional herbal formulae

Allergy Research	Phyllanthus Complex (incl Milk Thistle)	1 at each meal

Specific Phase II support formula

Allergy Research	Thiodox	1 tablet with breakfast & dinner

Liver Support Plan – Lower Phase I than II

(When this has been proved by a liver detox test)

Multi-nutrient formula

Allergy Research	Fast & Be Clear Powder	1 tsp in water twice daily for 3 days, then 2 tsp in water twice daily for 3 days with or away from food, then 3 tsp in water

twice daily for 3 days, then 1 scoop twice daily thereafter

Specific Phase I support formula

Biotics Research	A.D.H.S.	1 at breakfast, 1 at lunch

Anti-Cravings Plan

Special calcium & co-factors formula found to reduce cravings

Allergy Research	XCravings powder	1 tsp in water or diluted juice on an empty stomach once to three times daily

A Note on Probiotics

Due to the fact that there are many different species of friendly bacteria within a healthy gut, it is recommended to rotate probiotics as time goes by. For those of you following a program which features *Lactobacillus* GG, please rotate the specific probiotic when it runs out with the following two items, in sequence:

Allergy Research	Bifido Biotics	2 with a meal per day
Allergy Research	*Lactobacillus plantarum, Rhamnosus, Salivarius*	2 with a meal per day

A Note on Fiber

Fiber can serve a number of benefits. It helps to smooth the transit of matter through your colon, and at the same time helps to carry out toxins. It also helps to hydrate the large intestine. If you are constipated or wish to soften your stools, take the supplement Colon Plus in addition to any of the above programs. Do not take the Colon Plus at the same time as you take any other supplement.

Biotics Research	Colon Plus	3 capsules in between meals with a large glass of water, once or twice daily

Colon Plus contains psyllium seed powder, mannitol, kelgin, apple pectin, peppermint leaf powder, vitamin C, anise, flax seed powder, bromelain, celery powder, *Lactobacillus acidophilus* (DDS-1), aloe vera powder, and prune powder.

The ingredients for all of these items are shown on the website: www.thefoodintolerancebible.com

You can obtain all of these supplements directly from suppliers' websites. See Appendix IV for more information.

Summary

You have now learned what you need to do to address your food intolerance(s). You have been given an outline of how to identify and tackle other conditions with remedial plans to hasten your progress, and in some cases achieve what could never be achieved through diet alone. I hope you will emerge all the healthier for having done so. You are now armed with guidelines about how to avoid food intolerances in the future as well as how to eat more healthily than before. Enjoy Antoinette's recipes. I wish you the best of health.

Part Four

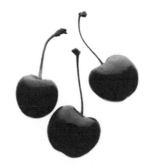

What Can I Eat?

16

Introduction to the Recipes

This collection of recipes features very quick and easy dishes, as well as those that are a little more time consuming. I hope that this will appeal both to working people with very limited time for entertaining and those juggling a demanding family life.

Now down to practicalities. There is now a wide range of gluten-free flour available, but not many will suit this particular book. You can mix your own blend to suit, depending on your dietary needs. Please take into consideration that each variety of flour has a different absorbency level and the amount of flour or liquid needed must therefore be adjusted accordingly. Sometimes you may have to add a little extra liquid if the mixture is too stiff or dry. If the mixture is too wet, you may need to add a fraction more flour. If you keep using the same brands or mix of flour, you will soon be able to judge this without a moment's thought.

Throughout the recipes, all solid ingredients are given in metric first, followed by American imperial and cup measurements. Liquid measurements are given in metric and cup measurements (1 cup = 8 fluid ounces). Please follow one set of measurements in each recipe, as they are not interchangeable. All recipes have been tested using each set of measurements.

Unless otherwise stated all tablespoon or teaspoon measures are level.

Organic products have been used in all the recipes but this I leave to your discretion. I have specified organic if the products have been easy to find but not if they have been unavailable at local superstores or health food stores. You'll find lots of helpful information at the back of the book with a contact address for the Whole Food Market® organization. If you are not familiar with a product used in the recipes, the list of what I keep on my kitchen shelves (on pages 170–1) or your local whole foods market (see page 325) should provide guidance.

When buying products, always check the label to ensure that the variety you buy is free of the allergens you are trying to avoid. In addition, before you begin any recipe, please look through it carefully to ensure that those who are going to eat it are tolerant of all the ingredients. You don't want to go to the trouble and expense of preparing a dish only to find that one of your guests is unable to eat it!

I hope that these little snippets of information will help make cooking and entertaining easy as well as rewarding.

Symbols

The symbols shown below are used throughout the recipes to enable you to judge their suitability. All the recipes are gluten free and therefore wheat free, so a wheat-free symbol is not included. Goat's products feature in a number of recipes but for most of these you can easily substitute rice or other suitable milks, cheeses or yogurts if you wish.

GF = Gluten free (which is wheat free)

LF = Lactose free (which is dairy free)

GO = Contains goat's products

V = Vegetarian (suitable for vegetarians but not vegans)

SF = Sugar free

SOF = Soya free

YF = Yeast free

NF = Nightshade free – i.e. no potatoes, tomatoes, eggplant, sweet peppers (bell peppers), chilies, blackcurrants

EF = Egg free

17

Useful Ingredients

My kitchen shelves positively groan with food and drink so that I never run short of anything. Here is a short list of the most useful ingredients and foods that you might like to have on your shelves, or in the refrigerator or freezer.

If you can buy organic produce and products whenever possible you will notice a great difference in the taste, texture, and quality of the finished recipe.

On the Shelves

Organic rice, quinoa and tapioca flour

Organic quinoa, amaranth, millet and rice flakes for granola

Gluten-free baking powder, bicarbonate of soda (baking soda), cream of tartar and arrowroot

Organic walnuts, pine nuts and hazelnuts, and ground, flaked and whole almonds

Organic sunflower, pumpkin and sesame seeds

Pure Madagascan vanilla extract and rose water

Organic dried apricots, figs, dates, golden raisins, raisins and currants

Cold pressed and organic extra virgin olive oil, sunflower, avocado oil, walnut and sesame oils

Unsweetened organic carrot juice and jars of organic unsweetened pumpkin puree

Organic ground spices, saffron strands and fresh ginger root

Organic dried herbs, fresh herbs and garlic

Canned clear consommé (beef and chicken)

Organic wild, brown, risotto and pudding rice

Orgran gluten-, egg- and yeast-free pasta shapes, spaghetti, lasagna and fettuccini (available by mail order or in many supermarkets

Orgran allergy-free All-purpose Crumbs

Organic canned chickpeas, cannellini beans, flageolets, water chestnuts and artichoke hearts

Canned reduced-fat coconut milk, cartons of coconut cream and unsweetened desiccated (shredded) coconut

Allergy-free bouillon powder

Agar flakes

Verjuice (available by mail order and from specialist sections of large supermarkets)

Unsweetened organic fruit juice

Furikake Japanese seasoning (available from Planet Organic mail order)

In the Refrigerator

Aside from all the usual fresh foods in the refrigerator, I keep a few essentials for my recipes:

Black olives in oil

Organic goat's milk, cream, yogurt and cheeses

Trex (white vegetable shortening)
Dairy-free vegetable margarine spread

In the freezer

I try not to keep much in the freezer because I prefer fresh food. I have
the following foods for convenience and emergencies:
Large organic chicken and turkey breasts or escalopes
Organic frozen vegetables
Wild salmon steaks, jumbo shrimp, crayfish tails and crab
Organic frozen summer berries and fruit mixtures

18

Recipes

List of Recipes

Soups

Vegetarian Dishes

Pasta

Seafood and Fish

Poultry and Game

Meat

Desserts

Breakfast and Afternoon treats

Soups

Fennel and White Bean Soup

Fennel has a refreshing, aniseed flavour that livens up the soft texture and gentle taste of the white beans, to give a perfectly balanced and warming soup.

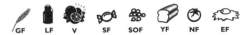

Serves 4–6

200g/7oz/1 cup organic butter beans soaked overnight in cold water,

drained and boiled in a pan of fresh water until soft or according

to the instructions on the package or 2 x 425g/15oz cans unsweetened

organic butter beans, drained and rinsed in cold running water

1 medium bulb organic fennel, trimmed and the fronds finely chopped for decoration

2 tablespoons organic cold pressed extra virgin olive oil

1 very large organic onion, finely diced

1 liter/4 cups strong allergy-free vegetable bouillon

Sea salt (optional) or freshly ground black pepper

First prepare the beans.

Finely slice the fennel bulb and stew, over gentle heat, with the oil and onions until the vegetables have softened. Add the beans, stir in the bouillon, bring to the boil and then simmer for about 25 minutes or until the vegetables are cooked through. Let the soup cool and, using a blender, process until smooth. Return the soup to the pan.

Season the soup to taste, sprinkle with the chopped fennel fronds and serve piping hot.

Ginger and Sweet Potato Soup

This delicious, Caribbean-style soup is full of exotic flavors and has a smooth silky texture. You can make it with fresh coconut and add chopped chilies if you can tolerate them on your diet.

Serves 6

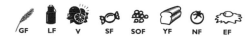

4 tablespoons organic cold pressed extra virgin olive oil

4 medium organic onions, finely chopped

2 large organic garlic cloves

2 large organic sweet potatoes, cubed

1 liter/4 cups allergy-free vegetable bouillon

250ml/1 cup coconut cream or organic coconut milk

5cm/2in piece peeled organic root ginger, coarsely chopped

Sea salt (optional) and freshly ground black pepper

2 heaped tablespoons chopped organic cilantro leaves

Heat the oil in a pan, stir in the onions and cook over medium heat until softened but not browned. Add the garlic, sweet potatoes, bouillon and coconut and bring to the boil. Cook for 20 minutes, stir in the ginger and cook for 10 minutes or until the potatoes are soft. Allow the soup to cool then process it using a blender. Return the soup to the pan, reheat and season to taste.

Serve sprinkled with the chopped cilantro.

Parsnip and Celeriac Soup

Celeriac makes a very useful alternative to potatoes – although it looks rather unappealing on the outside, once cooked, it is easily transformed into a light, fluffy mash or a creamy gratin Dauphinoise.

Serves 6

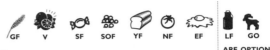

GF   V   SF   SOF   YF   NF   EF   LF   GO

ARE OPTIONAL

750ml/3 cups organic rice milk or goat's milk

750ml/3 cups allergy-free vegetable bouillon

2 medium or 340g/12oz/2½ cups peeled and cubed organic parsnips

1 small or 425g/15oz/2½ cups peeled and cubed organic celeriac

1 large organic garlic clove

3 large or 6 small cardamom pods, husks discarded

Sea salt (optional) and freshly ground black pepper

Place the milk and bouillon in a pan, add the cubed vegetables, garlic and cardamom seeds and bring to the boil over medium heat. Reduce the heat and simmer until the vegetables are soft. Let the soup cool and, using a blender, process the soup to a smooth purée. Return the soup to the pan and reheat but do not boil. Season to taste and serve.

Chilled Zucchini and Mint Soup

Cucumber is the traditional choice for chilled summer soup but for this recipe I have used zucchini, which give a creamy but light soup, flecked with the dark green of the skin. Chill the soup for 3 to 4 hours for best results.

Serves 4–6

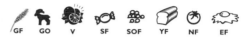

500g/1lb 2oz/4 cups medium-sized organic zucchini, trimmed and roughly chopped

750ml/3 cups strong allergy-free vegetable bouillon

500ml/2 cups plain unsweetened organic goat's yogurt

2 heaped tablespoons chopped fresh organic mint

2 heaped tablespoons chopped fresh organic parsley

2 trimmed organic scallions, sliced

1 small organic garlic clove

Sea salt (optional) and freshly ground black pepper

Optional

Crushed ice cubes (use filtered water) and chopped fresh organic mint leaves to serve

Put the zucchini and bouillon in a pan. Bring to the boil and cook over medium heat for 10 minutes. Remove the pan from the heat and leave until the mixture is cold. Process the soup in a blender with the yogurt, mint, parsley, scallions and garlic.

Transfer the soup to a serving bowl, season to taste and chill until needed. Just before serving, stir in crushed ice cubes and fresh mint.

Minestrone Soup

This traditional Italian soup has come back into fashion over the last few years thanks to the chefs at various trendy restaurants. You can make it with any leftover vegetables or pasta, which makes it cheap and versatile.

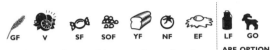

GF   V   SF   SOF   YF   NF   EF | LF   GO
ARE OPTIONAL

Serves 6

115g/4oz/1cup organic cannellini beans, soaked overnight in cold water, drained and
cooked in fresh water for about 1hr or according to instructions on the packet or use 2 x 255g/
9oz cans sugar-free organic cooked beans, rinsed

2 tablespoons organic cold pressed extra virgin olive oil and a little extra for drizzling

2 medium-sized organic carrots, finely chopped

1 large organic red onion, finely chopped

3 sticks organic celery, finely chopped

2–3 large organic garlic cloves, finely chopped

155g/5½ oz/1½ cups fresh organic spring greens, tough stalks discarded, leaves finely shredded

1.5 liters/6 cups allergy-free strong vegetable bouillon

A few sprigs fresh organic thyme

About 8 large organic sage leaves, shredded

A good handful organic parsley, finely chopped

Sea salt (optional) and freshly ground black pepper

A pinch of organic ground cloves

100g/3½ oz/1 cup cooked allergy-free pasta (penne, farfalle, macaroni, etc.)

Optional
Freshly grated hard organic goat's cheese to serve

First prepare the beans.

Heat the oil in a large pan, add the carrots, onion and celery and cook gently until softened. Add the cooked, drained and rinsed cannellini beans, garlic and spring greens and cook for a couple of minutes. Stir in the bouillon, thyme leaves, sage, parsley, seasoning and cloves, bring to the boil and simmer for about 20 minutes or until all the vegetables are tender. Stir in the cooked pasta, adjust the seasoning and serve sprinkled with the grated cheese, if using.

Smooth Carrot and Rice Soup

This soup is my version of healthy comfort food for cold days or days when you're feeling delicate and need something warm and gentle on the stomach.

Serves 4–6

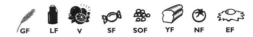

1 large organic onion, finely chopped

750g/1lb 10oz/6 cups peeled organic carrots, finely chopped

2 tablespoons organic cold pressed extra virgin olive oil

1.25 litres/5 cups allergy-free vegetable bouillon

1 teaspoon fresh organic tarragon leaves or ½ teaspoon dried

3 heaped tablespoons organic short-grain white rice

Sea salt (optional) and freshly ground black pepper

2 heaped tablespoons freshly chopped organic parsley

Gently cook the onion and carrots together in the oil until softened but not browned. Add the bouillon, tarragon and rice, bring to the boil, reduce heat to medium and simmer the soup for about 30 minutes or until the rice and vegetables are cooked through. When the soup is cool, process in a blender until smooth. Reheat the soup, season according to taste and serve hot, sprinkled with the chopped parsley.

Vegetarian Dishes

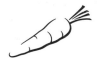

Spicy Parsnip and Leek Purée

Parsnips have an affinity with spices and there is another recipe using this combination on page 197. Serve the purée with other vegetarian dishes or – if you eat meat – roast, grilled or cold meats, game or chicken.

Serves 4

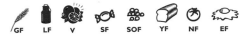

GF   LF   V   SF   SOF   YF   NF   EF

680g/1½ lb/5 cups organic parsnips, peeled and cut into chunks

55g/2oz/¼ cup dairy-free vegetable margarine spread

1 organic garlic clove, crushed

1 teaspoon ground organic coriander

1 teaspoon ground organic cumin

2 organic leeks, trimmed and thinly sliced

1 tablespoon chopped fresh organic cilantro or parsley leaves

Sea salt (optional) and freshly ground black pepper

Cook the parsnips in a pan of boiling water until tender. Meanwhile, melt the margarine in a skillet, add the garlic, spices and leeks and cook gently until soft.

Drain the parsnips and process to a coarsely mashed consistency in a food processor. Add the leek mixture, season generously, stir in the fresh cilantro or parsley, purée to a smoother consistency and serve immediately.

Peach, Spinach and Pistachio Salad

A drizzle of nut oil can make virtually any salad special enough for a dinner or lunch party, so why not try different ones? You can make this salad using nectarines instead of peaches and, in winter, with ripe pears cut into quarters or thick slices.

Serves 4

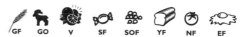

4 small handfuls trimmed fresh organic spinach leaves, washed and drained

4 small ripe organic peaches, peeled and cut into thick slices

55g/2oz/⅓ cup shelled pistachio nuts or more if you want

100–150g/3½–5oz/⅔ cup mild and creamy soft organic goat's cheese

1 tablespoon organic walnut oil

2 tablespoons organic cold pressed extra virgin olive oil or more if desired

Sea salt (optional) and freshly ground black pepper

About 16 fresh organic basil leaves, shredded

1 tablespoon Verjuice

Arrange the spinach leaves on each plate and place the peach slices on top. Scatter the salad with the nuts and little blobs of goat's cheese. I use a teaspoon and clean fingers for this.

In a small bowl, mix the oils together with the salt (optional), pepper, basil and Verjuice and whisk vigorously. Spoon the dressing over the peach salads and serve immediately.

Chicory, Red Onion and White Bean Salad

This salad can be eaten as a simple lunch with allergy-free bread or an allergy-free pasta salad. Alternatively, it makes an excellent accompaniment to broiled game or oily fish.

Serves 4–6

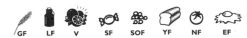

200g/7oz/1 cup dried organic butter beans, soaked overnight in cold water, rinsed and cooked in boiling water for about 1 hour or according to the instructions on the packet or 2 x 395g/14oz cans unsweetened organic butter beans, drained

1 small organic red onion, finely chopped

24 large pitted black olives in oil (not vinegar), drained and halved

2 tablespoons chopped organic basil leaves

1 organic garlic clove, crushed

Sea salt (optional) and freshly ground black pepper

1 tablespoon avocado oil

2 tablespoons organic cold pressed extra virgin olive oil

2 tablespoons Verjuice

2 large heads organic Belgian endive, trimmed, cut lengthways into 8 pieces and separated

2 tablespoons finely chopped fresh organic parsley

Prepare the beans first.

Drain the beans, rinse under cold running water and shake dry. In a serving bowl, mix the beans with the onion, olives, basil, garlic, seasoning, both the oils and the Verjuice. Toss the Belgian endive leaves with the beans until well coated and serve the salad sprinkled with chopped parsley.

Moroccan Carrot Salad

Raw carrots may be wonderfully healthy but it can get a bit boring if you simply chomp away on them straight out of the bag. This very easy recipe makes raw carrots a bit more interesting, and is great with any Indian or Eastern-type meals.

Serves 6

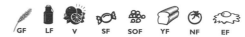

600g/1lb 5oz/5 cups organic carrots, peeled and coarsely grated

2 large organic garlic cloves, crushed

4 tablespoons cold pressed extra virgin olive oil

2 tablespoons Verjuice

2 teaspoons organic cumin seed

Sea salt (optional) and freshly ground black pepper

2 heaped tablespoons chopped fresh organic cilantro leaves

To serve

1 or 2 heaped tablespoons chopped fresh organic herbs – cilantro leaves, chives, basil or parsley are all delicious

Mix all the ingredients, in the given order, in a serving bowl. Just before serving, sprinkle the carrot salad with the extra herbs and serve or chill until needed.

Onion and Goat's Cheese Tarts

I love easy and relaxed recipes that you can alter as the feeling or season takes you. In summer, I make toppings from whatever vegetables I have a glut of; in winter, anchovies and olives make delicious alternatives.

Serves 6

GF   GO   V   SF   SOF   YF   NF   EF

Pastry

30g/1oz/scant ¼ cup organic tapioca flour

30g/1oz/scant ¼ cup organic quinoa flour

170g/6oz/1¼ cups organic rice flour

70g/2½ oz/⅓ cup pure vegetable shortening

70g/2½ oz/⅓ cup dairy-free vegetable margarine spread

A pinch of fine salt (optional)

Cold filtered water

Filling

1 large organic onion, halved and very thinly sliced

2 tablespoons organic cold pressed extra virgin olive oil

Sea salt (optional) and freshly ground black pepper

1 heaped tablespoon dairy-free vegetable margarine spread

2 heaped tablespoons organic rice flour

250ml/1 cup organic goat's or rice milk

100g/3½ oz/¾ cup grated hard organic goat's cheese

100g/3½ oz/½ cup chopped medium-soft organic goat's cheese

Topping

A sprinkling of organic pine nuts

25.5cm/10in round, loose-bottomed, fluted tart pan

Preheat the oven to 200°C/400°F.

Make the pastry in a food processor. Mix the flours, shortening, margarine and salt (optional) together until the mixture resembles breadcrumbs. Add a little water at a time and mix briefly until the pastry comes together into a wet ball of dough.

Roll out the pastry on a floured surface into a slightly larger circle than the base of the pan. Use the rolling pin to guide the pastry into the pan and clean fingers to gently mold and push the pastry up the sides of it. Prick the base with a fork and neaten the edges. Bake the pastry blind for about 15 minutes until just golden at the edges.

Meanwhile, gently fry the onions in the oil, in a large saucepan, until they are soft but not browned. Season with salt (optional) and pepper and transfer the mixture to a plate. Using the same pan, gently heat the margarine and then stir in the flour. Gradually add the milk, stirring constantly to give a smooth white sauce. When the sauce is thick and has reached boiling point, stir in the grated cheese and then the onions.

Gently stir the goat's cheese into the onion sauce and then fill the pastry with the onion mixture. Cover with pine nuts and bake in the oven for about 20 minutes or until golden and bubbling.

Cool slightly, then carefully lift the tart, still on its base, out of the pan and place it on a plate to serve.

Roast Vegetable Salad with Melted Goat's Cheese

Mediterranean vegetables taste sweeter when roasted with olive oil and a little seasoning. Throughout the seasons, you can experiment with different goat's cheeses and use different herbs.

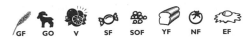

Serves 4

2 large organic zucchini, trimmed and cut into fairly large wedges

2 large or 3 very small bulbs of organic fennel, trimmed and cut into fairly large wedges

170g/6oz/1 cup organic trimmed asparagus, any tough ends removed or about 8 organic baby leeks, trimmed enough to fit onto your serving plates

1 large organic red onion, trimmed and cut into eight wedges

6 tablespoons organic cold pressed extra virgin olive oil

2 organic garlic cloves, finely sliced

Sea salt (optional) and freshly ground black pepper

4 thick slices of any kind of firm round goat's cheese with rind, approximately 55g/2oz each

2 tablespoons Verjuice

Fresh organic basil leaves, shredded

Preheat the oven to 220°C/425°F.

Mix all the vegetables together in a large non-stick roasting pan with the oil, garlic, plenty of salt (optional) and pepper and roast them for about 25 minutes until softened and tinged with golden brown. Turn all the vegetables over and roast for another 15 minutes or until cooked through.

Place the slices of cheese on top of the vegetables, ensuring they are spaced well enough apart so that you can easily transfer them, with a portion of vegetables, onto four warmed serving plates.

Roast the cheese and vegetables for about 5 minutes until just melted then quickly transfer onto the plates and serve sprinkled with the Verjuice and basil leaves.

Avocado and Hummus Dip

This delicious combination is an even healthier recipe than the usual guacamole or plain hummus. A large dollop of this dip on a salad or on top of a baked sweet potato is great for a lunchtime snack.

Serves 4–6

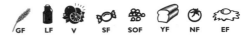

395g/14oz can organic chickpeas (check label for dietary requirements) or

115g/4oz/⅔ cup organic chickpeas soaked in cold water overnight, drained and rinsed, boiled in water for about 1hr or until cooked through

1 teaspoon organic sesame oil

4 tablespoons organic cold pressed extra virgin olive oil

2 ripe organic avocados, peeled and coarsely chopped

1 large organic garlic clove

Sea salt (optional) and freshly ground black pepper

2 tablespoons Verjuice

15g/½ oz/¼ cup fresh organic cilantro, trimmed

Drain and rinse the cooked chickpeas under cold running water. Put the chickpeas, oils, chopped avocado, garlic, seasoning, Verjuice and cilantro together in a food processor and whiz until just smooth. Scrape around the bowl, adjust the seasoning and whiz briefly again.

Transfer to a serving bowl, cover and chill until needed.

Flageolet, Avocado and Pine Nut Salad

Here is another easy salad that can be served any time of year. It's great served with other vegetarian salads or with cold meats, chicken or fish.

Serves 4–6

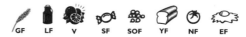

170g/6oz/1 cup organic flageolets, soaked overnight in cold water, drained and cooked for about 1hr or until cooked through or 2 x 310g/11oz cans organic unsweetened flageolets, drained and rinsed under cold running water

½ large or 1 small organic red onion, finely chopped

2 ripe organic avocados, chopped and sprinkled with 2 tablespoons of Verjuice

55g/2oz/⅓ cup organic pine nuts, toasted until golden

2 heaped tablespoons chopped organic flat leaf parsley

2 tablespoons organic cold pressed extra virgin olive oil

2 tablespoons avocado oil

1 organic garlic clove, crushed

Sea salt (optional) and freshly ground pepper

Drain and rinse the beans under cold running water and then combine all the ingredients together in a serving dish. Adjust the seasoning to taste and serve.

Quinoa Risotto

Risotto made with quinoa has a delicious flavor and a lovely texture – the grains absorb all the flavours but remain separated and crunchy. This recipe is the perfect accompaniment to the Lamb Kebabs on page 252.

Serves 4

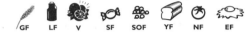

170g/6oz/1 cup organic quinoa

2 teaspoons dairy-free vegetable margarine spread

2 teaspoons organic sunflower oil

1 organic red onion, finely chopped

2 organic garlic cloves, crushed

2 teaspoons chopped organic marjoram leaves

About 300g/10oz/2 cups mixed chopped organic vegetables of your choice

750ml/3 cups boiling allergy-free bouillon

Sea salt (optional) and freshly ground black pepper

4 tablespoons chopped fresh organic parsley

Place the quinoa in a colander, rinse under cold running water for a minute and set aside.

Heat the margarine and oil gently in a pan, add the onion and cook until softened. Stir in the garlic, marjoram and vegetables and cook for a couple of minutes before adding the quinoa, bouillon, seasoning and half the parsley.

Simmer the risotto for 20 minutes, adding a little water if the mixture becomes dry before it is cooked through. When all the liquid is absorbed, leave the risotto to sit for 5 minutes, then fluff up with a fork and adjust the seasoning to taste. Serve immediately, sprinkled with the remaining parsley.

Spiced Parsnip and Mixed Leaf Salad

This delicious warm salad can be served as an appetizer, part of a buffet or simply as an accompaniment to other vegetarian salads.

Serves 6

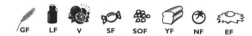

2 heaped teaspoons organic cumin seeds

2 heaped teaspoons organic ground coriander

½ teaspoon organic ground turmeric

Sea salt (optional) and freshly ground black pepper

200ml/¾ cup coconut cream

2 tablespoons organic cold pressed extra virgin olive oil and a little extra for drizzling

1kg/2lb 4oz/7cups medium-sized organic parsnips, trimmed, peeled, halved horizontally and cut into even-sized lengths

135g/4½ oz pack or 6 handfuls mixed prepared organic arugula, baby spinach or other salad leaves

Preheat the oven to 200°C/400°F/.

In a bowl, mix all the spices and seasoning with the coconut cream and oil.

Cook the parsnips in boiling water until softened. Drain, refresh them under cold running water and leave them for 5 minutes in the colander. Put the parsnips into a large roasting dish so that they lie in a single layer. Pour the spice mixture over the parsnips and toss until they are well coated.

Roast the parsnips for about 50 minutes to an hour, depending on size. They should be golden and crispy on both sides. Place the parsnips on top of the salad leaves, drizzle with a little extra oil and serve immediately.

Griddled Zucchini with Mint

If you don't already possess a griddle, I suggest investing in the largest one possible so that you can griddle enough to serve four people at a time. You can place it over two of the rings on your stove-top. Always heat the griddle until very hot before you start cooking and don't pour oil on the griddle – oil the food lightly instead or even cook with no oil at all.

Serves 4

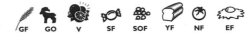

4 large organic zucchini

Sea salt (optional) and freshly ground black pepper

Organic cold pressed extra virgin olive oil

200g/7oz/1cup feta cheese made from goat's milk, crumbled or chopped

4 tablespoons chopped fresh organic mint leaves

Slice the zucchini lengthwise and sprinkle with salt (optional). Leave for 15 minutes and then rinse off with cold running water and pat dry with paper towels. Heat the griddle until very hot, brush the zucchini with oil and griddle until charred lines are visible on both sides and the vegetables are just cooked through.

Arrange the zucchini in a serving dish, season with salt (optional) and pepper, drizzle with plenty of oil, scatter with the cheese and mint leaves and toss to combine.

Serve or cover and keep cool until needed.

Watermelon, Walnut and Feta Salad

This bright and cheerful salad is ideal as an appetizer before a barbecue or as part of a selection of salads for a party. We often have this salad for lunch with warm bread dipped in a dark, fruity olive oil.

Serves 6

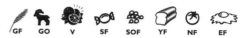

½ medium-sized ripe watermelon, skin removed and flesh cut into bite-size cubes

85g/3oz/¾ cup walnut pieces, coarsely chopped

200g/7oz/1 cup feta cheese made from goat's milk, crumbled or cubed

15g/½ oz/1 cup freshly chopped organic mint leaves

2 tablespoons organic cold pressed extra virgin olive oil

2 tablespoons organic walnut oil

Freshly ground black pepper

Put the chopped up watermelon, walnuts, cheese and mint in a large salad bowl. Mix the oils and pepper into the salad and serve. You can chill the salad for a few hours but after that it becomes a bit watery.

Asparagus Mousse with Herb Dressing

These little mousses are wonderfully light and perfect for summer eating. You can serve them as an appetizer for eight or allow two per person, set them on a large bed of salad and serve as a main course.

Serves 4–8

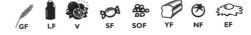

GF   LF   V   SF   SOF   YF   NF   EF

Herb dressing

2 heaped tablespoons chopped fresh organic herbs of your choice – parsley, basil, dill, cilantro, chives or a mixture of two varieties

2 tablespoons Verjuice

4 tablespoons organic cold pressed extra virgin olive oil

Asparagus Mousse

750g/1lb 10oz/4¼ cups fresh organic asparagus

2 heaped tablespoons agar flakes

Sea salt (optional) and freshly ground black pepper

Pinch of organic nutmeg

250ml/1 cup allergy-free vegetable bouillon

A couple of handfuls of mixed baby salad leaves

8 small ramekins lined with plastic wrap or non-stick tin molds

First check that the plastic food wrap lining the ramekins has enough of an overhang to fold over what will be the base of the mousse.

Now make the dressing by beating the herbs, Verjuice and oil together in a bowl. Transfer to a small pouring jug.

Cut off the tough lower third of each asparagus spear and discard. Poach the asparagus in boiling water until soft, drain over a large measuring jug and retain 500ml/2 cups of the liquid. Reserve 8 asparagus tips for decoration, chop up the remaining asparagus and place in a food processor with half the reserved liquid. Blend until smooth.

Put the remaining liquid into a small saucepan and sprinkle with the agar flakes. Place over medium heat and simmer for about 2 minutes or until the flakes have dissolved. Stir and simmer for another 2 minutes. Cool slightly, add to the asparagus purée in the food processor and blend until smooth. Season the mixture to taste with salt (optional), pepper and nutmeg.

Pour the mixture into the prepared ramekins, cover with the plastic wrap and chill in the refrigerator until set, which should be within 4 hours.

To turn each mousse out, peel back the plastic wrap, hold the ramekin over the plate and give it a firm shake and thump on the base. Surround the mousse/s with a few mixed leaves and drizzle with the dressing. Place one of the cooked asparagus tips on top of each mousse and serve.

Pasta

Tagliatelle with Seafood

I am so relieved that you can buy so many different styles of allergy-free pasta now – and that they're available in lots of good supermarkets. It means we no longer need to trek to a health food store for such an indispensable foodstuff.

Serves 2–3

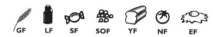

115g/4oz/½ cup shelled organic baby fava beans

170g/6oz/2 cups allergy-free tagliatelle or spaghetti

4 tablespoons organic cold pressed extra virgin olive oil

395g/14oz/4⅔ cups frozen seafood mix – mussels, scallops, shrimp, squid etc.

1–2 organic garlic cloves, crushed

1 tablespoon finely chopped fresh organic dill

1 heaped tablespoon chopped fresh organic parsley

Sea salt (optional) and freshly ground black pepper

Cook the fava beans in a small pan of boiling water until tender and then drain them. If the skins are soft they can be left on; if they are tough they should be peeled off and discarded.

Bring a pan of salted (optional) water to the boil, add the pasta and cook until slightly softened. Drain and rinse the pasta under cold water. Refill the pan with boiling water, return the pasta to the pan and cook until al dente. This method prevents the pasta becoming too sticky.

Heat the oil in a pan over moderate heat, add the fava beans, seafood and garlic and briefly sauté. Add the dill and parsley and shake the pan over the heat.

Drain the pasta and toss with the seafood mixture in a warm serving bowl. Season to taste and serve immediately.

Macaroni Cheese

Goat's milk and cheese impart a delicious, rich flavor to a dish that is a favorite of children and adults alike.

Serves 4–6

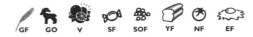

750ml/3 cups organic goat's milk

Sea salt (optional) and freshly ground black pepper

2 organic bay leaves

½ an organic onion studded with 4 cloves

Plenty of freshly grated organic nutmeg

255g/9oz/3 cups allergy-free macaroni

55g/2oz/¼ cup dairy-free vegetable margarine spread

3 heaped tablespoons organic rice flour

115g/4oz/1 cup hard organic goat's cheese, grated

Put the milk, salt (optional), pepper, bay leaves, clove-studded onion and nutmeg in a pan and heat slowly until it reaches boiling point. Remove from the heat and leave to infuse for 20 minutes.

Bring a pan of salted (optional) water to the boil, add the pasta and cook until slightly softened. Drain and rinse the pasta, refill the pan with boiling water, return the pasta to the pan and cook until al dente. This method prevents it becoming too sticky.

Drain the milk into a pouring jug and discard the other ingredients.

Melt the margarine in a large, non-stick pan over low heat. Stir in the flour and, beating until smooth, gradually incorporate the flavored milk. The sauce will be thick and smooth by the time it reaches boiling point. Cook for a further minute and then stir in 85g/3oz of the cheese. Adjust the seasoning to taste and stir in the macaroni.

Spoon the mixture into a heatproof serving dish, sprinkle with the remaining cheese – or more if you like – and broil until golden and bubbling.

If you make the dish in advance, you can keep it covered and cool and then reheat it in a very hot oven until golden and bubbling.

Rigatoni, Olives and Roast Squash

Roasting squash intensifies its sweet flavor but if you don't have time for this you can gently sauté it in a pan. Try different squashes in season and see which you like best.

Serves 4–6

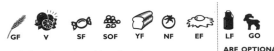

GF   V   SF   SOF   YF   NF   EF   LF   GO

ARE OPTIONAL

1 organic butternut squash, halved, seeded, peeled and cut into bite-size pieces

6 tablespoons organic cold pressed extra virgin olive oil

Sea salt (optional) and freshly ground black pepper

1 heaped teaspoon finely chopped organic rosemary

340g/12oz/4 cups allergy-free rigatoni or other similar-shaped pasta

10 large organic sage leaves, finely chopped

About 24 large, pitted black olives in oil not vinegar

1 large organic garlic clove, crushed

2 tablespoons finely chopped fresh organic parsley

Optional

Plenty of freshly grated hard organic goat's cheese

Preheat the oven to 220°C/425°F.

Toss the pieces of squash in half the oil, place on a non-stick baking tray and sprinkle with salt (optional), pepper and rosemary. Roast the squash in the oven until tender, which will be about 40 minutes depending on size.

Meanwhile, bring a pan of salted (optional) water to the boil, add the pasta and cook until slightly softened. Drain and rinse the pasta, refill the pan with boiling water, return the pasta to the pan and cook until al dente. This method prevents it becoming too sticky. Drain the pasta and transfer it to a warm serving bowl.

Briefly heat the remaining oil in a small pan over medium heat. Add the sage, olives and garlic and toss together for about a minute. Mix the sage oil and the squash into the pasta and adjust the seasoning. Serve sprinkled with the chopped parsley.

Spaghetti and Meatballs

This pasta recipe if always a firm favorite with the children and is easy and filling. These meatballs are made with lamb but you can use organic beef for a change.

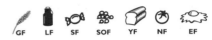

Serves 4

Sauce

2 tablespoons organic cold pressed extra virgin olive oil and a little extra for cooking the meatballs

1 large organic onion, halved and finely chopped

3 organic celery sticks, tough strings removed, finely chopped

1 organic leek, trimmed, tough outer layers removed, finely chopped

1 teaspoon fresh or dried organic oregano

2 organic bay leaves

1 large organic garlic clove, crushed

500ml/2 cups organic carrot juice

Sea salt (optional) and freshly ground black pepper

125ml/½ cup organic unsweetened pumpkin purée

Meatballs

595g/1lb 5oz lean organic minced (ground) lamb

10–12 fresh organic sage leaves, finely chopped

2 organic garlic cloves, crushed

To serve

340–400g/12–14oz/4–5 cups allergy-free spaghetti

Chopped fresh organic parsley or basil

First, make the sauce. Heat the oil in a large pan, add the onions and cook over moderate heat until softened. Add the chopped celery and leek and continue to cook gently until the vegetables are golden at the edges. Stir in the oregano, bay leaves and garlic and cook for a few minutes.

Stir in the carrot juice, salt (optional) and pepper and simmer the sauce for about 20 minutes. Mix in the pumpkin purée and allow the mixture to cool.

Purée the sauce in a blender, return it to the pan to heat through, and adjust the seasoning.

Mix all the meatball ingredients in a bowl and, taking about a walnut-size piece at a time, mould the mixture with your hands into about 20 balls. Set the meatballs aside.

Bring a pan of salted (optional) water to the boil, add the spaghetti and cook until slightly softened, separating it with a fork from time to time. Drain and rinse the spaghetti in running water, return it to the pan and cook until al dente in fresh boiling water. This method prevents the pasta becoming sticky.

Meanwhile, heat a drizzle of oil in a large non-stick skillet, add the meatballs and sauté until cooked through and golden brown. Pour in the sauce and reheat together, over a low heat, while you drain the cooked pasta.

Transfer the drained pasta to a warm serving bowl and top with the meatballs and sauce. Serve sprinkled with chopped parsley or basil.

Salmon Lasagna

Salmon labeled 'wild' roams the sea freely and catches its own food of crustaceans, which is why it is an orange color. At the time of writing this, wild salmon from Alaska were plentiful and available in many good supermarkets and fishmongers.

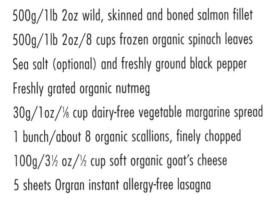

Serves 4

500g/1lb 2oz wild, skinned and boned salmon fillet

500g/1lb 2oz/8 cups frozen organic spinach leaves

Sea salt (optional) and freshly ground black pepper

Freshly grated organic nutmeg

30g/1oz/⅛ cup dairy-free vegetable margarine spread

1 bunch/about 8 organic scallions, finely chopped

100g/3½ oz/½ cup soft organic goat's cheese

5 sheets Orgran instant allergy-free lasagna

Cheese sauce

55g/2oz/¼ cup dairy-free margarine spread

3 heaped tablespoons organic rice flour

625–750ml/2½–3 cups organic rice or goat's milk

140g/5oz/¼ cup freshly grated hard organic goat's cheese

Preheat the oven to 190°C/375°F.

Slice the salmon into bite-size strips.

Cook the spinach in a non-stick pan, over low heat, until the water has evaporated and the spinach has thawed completely. Spread half the spinach over the base of a lasagne dish and season with salt (optional), pepper and nutmeg. Cover the spinach with the salmon strips.

Melt the margarine in a pan, add the scallions, fry over medium heat until softened and then spoon the mixture over the fish. Dot the salmon with little dollops of soft cheese.

Now make the cheese sauce. Melt the margarine in a non-stick pan over medium heat and stir in the flour. Beat until smooth, gradually adding the rice or goat's milk. When the sauce is thick and reaches boiling point, stir in half the grated cheese, salt (optional), pepper and plenty of grated nutmeg. Remove the sauce from the heat.

Cover the salmon mixture with a criss-cross arrangement of lasagna. Cover the lasagne with the remaining spinach, ensuring that the edges and corners are covered. Top with the cheese sauce.

Sprinkle the remaining grated cheese over the top and bake in the oven for about 40 minutes if you have followed the instructions on the packet of lasagna and dipped it in boiling water for 1 minute. If you haven't done this then allow longer.

Tortelli with Walnuts and Basil

People are often surprised when they see nuts in pasta dishes but this is an every-day occurrence in Italy. Nuts add a lovely crunchy texture to dishes and, along with nut oils, provide essential oils for our bodies. Tortelli pasta swells up so much that the usual portion ratio does not apply, but if you use other pasta shapes you may need to use 170g/6oz/2 cups.

Serves 2

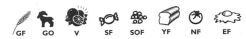

115g/4oz/1¼ cups allergy-free tortelli pasta (use bows or spirals if unavailable)

115g/4oz/1½ cups organic dwarf beans, topped, tailed and halved horizontally

1 organic garlic clove, crushed

3 tablespoons organic walnut oil

100g/3½ oz/½ cup organic semi-soft goat's cheese, roughly chopped or crumbled

Sea salt (optional) and freshly ground black pepper

55g/2oz/½ cup shelled organic walnut pieces

2 tablespoons shredded fresh organic basil leaves

Optional
Freshly grated hard goat's cheese for serving

Bring a pan of salted (optional) water to the boil, add the pasta and cook until slightly softened. Drain and refresh under cold water. Fill the pan with boiling water, return the pasta to the pan and cook until al dente. This method helps prevent the pasta becoming sticky.

Meanwhile, cook the beans until al dente in another pan of boiling water. Drain the beans, toss them back in the pan with the garlic and oil and cook, over low heat, for a couple of minutes. Drain the pasta. Toss the pasta with the beans and oil mixture in a warm serving bowl. Toss in the semi-soft goat's cheese, seasoning, walnuts and basil and serve immediately with or without extra grated cheese.

Fettuccini with Crab

Although I would always recommend you use fresh crab in season, out of season you can use a high-quality canned crab – but do check the label to make sure that there are no unsuitable ingredients. Otherwise use frozen crab meat or buy extra dressed crabs in season and freeze them yourself.

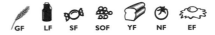

Serves 2

170g/6oz/2 cups allergy-free fettuccini

Sea salt (optional) and freshly ground black pepper

1 teaspoon organic sesame oil

2 tablespoons organic cold pressed extra virgin olive oil

1 teaspoon freshly grated organic root ginger

½ organic garlic clove, crushed

½ stick trimmed lemon grass, finely chopped

3 small organic scallions, trimmed and finely chopped

170g/6oz/1cup fresh, frozen (defrosted) or canned white crab meat

2 heaped tablespoons chopped fresh organic cilantro leaves

Bring a pan of salted (optional) water to the boil, add the pasta and cook until slightly softened. Drain and refresh under cold water. Fill the pan with boiling water, return the pasta to the pan and cook until al dente. This method prevents the pasta becoming sticky.

A few minutes before the end of the pasta cooking time, heat both the oils in a wok, add the ginger, garlic, lemon grass and scallions and stir-fry for a minute or two over high heat. Reduce the heat to low, toss in the crab and keep tossing until the crab has warmed through.

Drain the pasta and toss with the crab mixture in a warm serving bowl. Adjust the seasoning and serve immediately, sprinkled with the cilantro.

Penne with Bolognese-style Sauce

This traditional and robust sauce is so popular all over Europe that I feel a tomato-free version is definitely needed. You can use any shape of pasta for this dish.

Serves 6

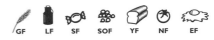

Bolognese sauce

4 tablespoons cold pressed extra virgin olive oil and extra for tossing the cooked pasta

1 large organic onion, finely chopped

1 large organic carrot, finely chopped

1 large stick organic celery, finely chopped

100g/3½ oz free-range chicken livers (from free-range chickens), any discolored or fatty bits discarded

2 large organic garlic cloves, crushed

455g/1lb organic lean ground beef

250ml/1 cup allergy-free chicken or vegetable bouillon

250ml/1 cup organic carrot juice

2 organic bay leaves

1 teaspoon fresh organic thyme leaves

1 teaspoon organic fennel seeds

Sea salt (optional) and freshly ground black pepper

3 heaped tablespoons unsweetened organic pumpkin purée to thicken the sauce

Pasta to serve

340–500g/12oz–1lb 2oz/4–5 cups allergy-free penne, depending on appetites

4 tablespoons freshly chopped organic parsley

Use a colander to rinse the chicken livers under cold running water. Leave them to drain and then roughly chop them.

Heat the oil in a large pan, add the vegetables, livers and garlic, cook for a few minutes and then stir in the beef. Cook for about 5 minutes, stirring from time to time. Add the bouillon, carrot juice, herbs and seasoning and simmer for about 40 minutes until tender. Ten minutes before the end of cooking time, stir the pumpkin purée into the sauce and simmer over slightly reduced heat until the sauce is thick.

Meanwhile, bring a pan of salted (optional) water to the boil, add the pasta and cook until slightly softened. Drain and refresh under cold water. Fill the pan with boiling water, return the pasta to the pan and cook until al dente. This method prevents it becoming sticky.

Drain the pasta and then toss in a warm serving bowl with the extra oil. Pour the bolognese sauce over the top and serve immediately, sprinkled with chopped parsley.

If you wish, you can double the quantities and freeze the sauce in smaller portions.

Chicken Livers, Fava Beans and Farfalle

This delicious pasta dish is best served with a mixed green leaf salad with herbs. If free-range or organic chicken livers are not available in your local supermarket, I suggest removing and freezing the chicken liver each time you cook a free-range or organic chicken.

Serves 4–6

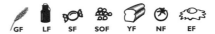

2 x 225g/8oz pack free-range or organic chicken livers, any discolored or fatty bits discarded

225g/8oz/1⅓ cups organic baby fava beans

340g/12oz/4 cups allergy-free farfalle (pasta bows)

4 tablespoons cold pressed extra virgin olive oil

2 organic garlic cloves, crushed

1 tablespoon fresh organic tarragon leaves, chopped

1 tablespoon dairy-free vegetable margarine spread

Sea salt (optional) and freshly ground black pepper

Plenty of freshly ground organic nutmeg

3 tablespoons freshly chopped organic chives

3 tablespoons freshly chopped organic parsley leaves

Rinse the chicken livers in cold running water and drain. Chop into bite-size pieces.

Bring a pan of water to the boil, add the fava beans and cook until al dente. Drain, rinse under cold water and leave to one side.

Bring a pan of salted (optional) water to the boil, add the pasta and cook until slightly softened. Drain and refresh under cold water. Fill the pan with boiling water, return the pasta to the pan and cook until al dente. This method helps prevent the pasta from becoming sticky.

A few minutes before the end of the pasta cooking time, heat the oil in a non-stick skillet over medium heat, add the chicken livers and sauté with the garlic. Once the livers are browned all over, add the fava beans, tarragon, margarine and seasoning and shake over the heat for a couple of minutes. The livers should be pink in the middle and golden brown on the outside.

Drain the pasta and toss in a warm serving bowl with the hot chicken liver mixture. Adjust the seasoning, dust with nutmeg and serve immediately, sprinkled with the chopped chives and parsley.

Spaghetti with Sage Oil

As I grow sage in my garden, we often have this simple dish for lunch. It only takes about 15 minutes from start to finish and while the pasta is cooking, you can put together a salad. It's also easy to double or triple the quantities if unexpected guests arrive.

Serves 2

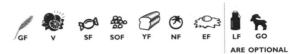

GF   V   SF   SOF   YF   NF   EF   LF   GO

ARE OPTIONAL

170g/6oz/2 cups allergy-free spaghetti

About 15g/½ oz/½ cup organic sage leaves, stems removed

4 tablespoons organic cold pressed extra virgin olive oil

1 organic garlic clove, crushed

Sea salt (optional) and freshly ground black pepper

Optional

Plenty of freshly grated hard organic goat's cheese to serve

Bring a pan of salted (optional) water to the boil, add the spaghetti and cook until slightly softened, separating the strands from time to time with a fork. Drain and rinse the pasta, return it to the pan, cover with fresh boiling water and cook until al dente. This method prevents the pasta becoming too sticky. Drain the pasta and transfer to a warm, heatproof serving bowl.

Meanwhile, shred the sage leaves. Heat the oil in a small pan until very hot but not smoking and throw in the sage leaves – beware, they will sizzle! After a few seconds throw in the garlic and sizzle for a few more seconds before tossing with the spaghetti. Season to taste and serve with or without the goat's cheese.

Seafood and Fish

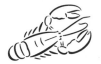

Smoked Mackerel Pâté

This pâté is always a good standby any time of the year and can be served with salads or allergy-free breads. Fresh horseradish is very hot, so beware!

Serves 4

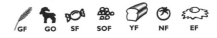

285g/10oz smoked organic mackerel fillets

A little freshly grated organic horseradish to taste

Sea salt (optional) and freshly ground black pepper

250ml/1 cup organic double goat's cream

Peel the skin off the mackerel fillets, break the fillets up and place in a food processor. Add the horseradish, salt (optional), pepper and cream and blend until smooth. Scrape round the sides of the bowl and adjust the seasoning if necessary before giving it a final blend. Scrape the pâté into a bowl and serve, or cover and chill until needed.

Stir-fried Shrimp

People with allergies can't just go to their local Chinese restaurant for take-out, so hopefully this recipe – which omits the usual problem ingredients – will be a welcome treat. It is a delicious combination of Japanese flavors and popular Asian ingredients.

Makes 4 small portions   [contains mushrooms] GF LF SF SOF YF NF   EF

225g/8oz/2 cups cooked shelled medium-sized shrimp

1 tablespoon organic rice flour mixed with 2 tablespoons Sanchi Furikake Japanese seasoning

1 tablespoon organic sesame oil

2 tablespoons organic cold pressed extra virgin olive oil

225g/8oz/4 cups organic tender-sweet cabbage, finely shredded

2 large organic garlic cloves, crushed

1 tablespoon freshly grated organic root ginger

170g/6oz/2 cups organic shiitake mushroom caps, sliced (or any combination of oriental mushrooms)

4 organic scallions, trimmed and finely shredded

Sea salt (optional) and freshly ground black pepper

15g/½ oz/½cup fresh organic cilantro leaves, chopped

On a small plate, toss the shrimp in the rice flour and Japanese seasoning mixture. Heat the oils in a wok or deep, non-stick skillet over high heat. Add the shrimp and cabbage and stir-fry for about 1 minute. Add the garlic, ginger, mushrooms and scallions and stir-fry for a few minutes until the shrimp are hot and the vegetables softened. Adjust the seasoning, adding more Japanese seasoning if you like.

   Sprinkle with the cilantro and serve immediately.

Roast Cod with Black Olive Crust

You can use any chunky white fish you like for this recipe. I usually serve this dish with a large salad of mixed leaves and herbs and a bowl of steamed wild and brown rice, sprinkled with plenty of freshly chopped parsley.

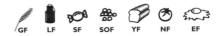

GF   LF   SF   SOF   YF   NF   EF

Serves 6

½ small organic onion, finely chopped

4 tablespoons cold pressed extra virgin olive oil plus extra for drizzling

1 large organic garlic clove, crushed

170g/6oz/1 cup pitted black olives in oil not vinegar, very finely chopped

55g/2oz/½ cup organic ground almonds

30g/1oz/¼ cup finely chopped organic almonds

Freshly ground black pepper and sea salt (optional)

6 x 170g/6oz cod or hoki fillets, boned and skinless

Preheat the oven to 200°C/400°F.

Make the olive topping first. Cook the onion in 3 tablespoons of oil until soft. Add the garlic and cook for another 2–3 minutes but do not let the ingredients burn. Mix the olives with the ground and chopped almonds, stir in the onion mixture and season to taste.

Place the fish fillets on a greased baking tray or sheet and brush with the remaining oil. Spoon the olive mixture on top of each fillet and press lightly. Bake in the oven for about 15 minutes, depending on the thickness of the fillets, then serve immediately.

Salmon on Celeriac Purée

Use wild salmon if you can, as its flavor and texture is far superior to that of mass-market farmed fish. The other downside of farmed fish is that because they don't eat a purely natural diet you can't be sure what you are actually eating.

Serves 4

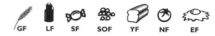

Celeriac purée

1 small organic celeriac, peeled and diced

1 tablespoon dairy-free vegetable margarine spread

Plenty of freshly grated organic nutmeg

Freshly grated black pepper and sea salt (optional)

Salmon

4 thick slices filleted wild salmon

1 tablespoon organic cold pressed extra virgin olive oil

1 teaspoon fresh organic thyme leaves

1 heaped tablespoon chopped fresh organic parsley or chives

Make the purée first. Cook the prepared celeriac until soft in a pan of boiling water. Drain the celeriac, return it to the pan and mash it until smooth. Stir in the margarine and nutmeg and season to taste.

Brush the salmon fillets with a little oil and season. Sprinkle them with thyme and cook the salmon under a hot broiler until opaque.

Spoon the celeriac purée onto the center of four warm plates and place the salmon at a jaunty angle on top. Serve immediately, topped with a sprinkling of parsley or chives.

Skate with Capers and Sage

Large, flat skate is ideal for frying – as it cooks, the pink-tinged flesh turns white and has a firm, meaty texture. The flesh easily flakes away from the gelatinous bones and melts in the mouth.

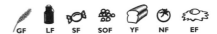

Serves 2

2 skate wings (whatever size you can eat!), rinsed under cold water

2 heaped tablespoons organic rice flour mixed with sea salt (optional) and

freshly ground black pepper

85g/3oz/⅓ cup dairy-free vegetable margarine spread

2 tablespoons capers in salt, washed and drained

6 large organic sage leaves, shredded

Pat the skate dry with paper towel. Put the seasoned flour on a plate and coat each skate wing evenly with the mixture. Melt the margarine in a non-stick skillet, add the skate and cook over medium heat until golden and cooked through. If the pan isn't big enough for both wings then cook them in two batches using half the margarine each time.

Remove the fish from the pan, transfer to a serving dish and keep warm. Cook the prepared capers and sage leaves for a few minutes in the pan.

Pour the juices, capers and sage over the skate wings and serve immediately.

Seared Squid with Arugula Pesto

Pesto made from arugula, rather than the more usual basil, has a lovely flavor. Your grocer should be happy to prepare the squid for you – ask him to clean and slice it up but keep the tentacles whole.

Serves 6

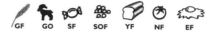

Pesto
30g/1oz/½ cup wild arugula leaves

2 organic garlic cloves, crushed

45g/1½ oz/⅓ cup finely grated hard organic goat's cheese

40g/1½ oz/¼ cup organic pine nuts

Sea salt (optional) and freshly ground black pepper

125ml/½ cup organic cold pressed extra virgin olive oil

Squid
Sea salt (optional) and freshly ground black pepper

900g/2lb prepared squid, rinsed in cold running water and drained, bodies sliced and tentacles trimmed

4 tablespoons organic cold pressed extra virgin olive oil

Make the pesto first. Put all the ingredients in a food processor and process briefly until you have a glossy sauce.

Season the squid with salt (optional) and pepper. Heat the oil in a large, non-stick pan over high heat, add the squid and sauté until golden. Serve immediately with the pesto drizzled over the top.

The squid and pesto is delicious served over allergy-free pasta or on a bed of steamed rice.

Spiced Swordfish with Salsa

If your supermarket doesn't have fresh swordfish, it is usually available frozen. You could also make this recipe with fresh tuna, which is more widely available.

Serves 4

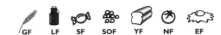

4 thick swordfish or tuna steaks

1 heaped tablespoon organic rice flour

2 tablespoons Furikake Japanese seasoning

Freshly ground black pepper

3 tablespoons organic cold pressed extra virgin olive oil

Avocado and Mango Salsa

1 large ripe organic avocado, diced

1 very small organic red onion, diced

1 small ripe organic mango, diced

Sea salt (optional) and freshly ground black pepper

4 tablespoons organic cold pressed extra virgin olive oil

4 tablespoons chopped organic basil or cilantro leaves

1 organic garlic clove, crushed

2 tablespoons Verjuice

Rinse the fish under cold water and drain for a few minutes. Combine the flour, Japanese seasoning and pepper on a plate and dust the fish steaks evenly with the mixture. Heat the oil in a skillet, add the fish and cook over medium heat until opaque and cooked through to your liking.

While the fish is cooking, make the salsa. Combine the diced avocado, onion and mango in a bowl and mix in the seasoning, oil, herbs, garlic and Verjuice. Transfer the salsa to a serving bowl and serve with the cooked fish.

Gray Mullet with Ginger and Scallions

On my way to catch the ferry from the Isle of Wight back to the U.K. mainland, I was taken to a wonderful traditional fishmonger tucked away down a winding lane. The gray mullet I bought had been freshly caught that morning and positively glistened with freshness. This simple recipe does justice to this delicious fish.

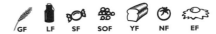

Serves 4–6

GF   LF   SF   SOF   YF   NF   EF

2 gray (or red) mullet (2 large ones if serving 6 people), cleaned and scaled

1 tablespoon organic sesame oil mixed with 2 tablespoons organic vegetable oil

Sea salt (optional) and freshly ground black pepper

8 organic scallions, very finely sliced

1 stick lemon grass, very finely sliced

1 heaped tablespoon finely grated organic root ginger

2 large organic garlic cloves, finely chopped

2 tablespoons chopped fresh organic cilantro leaves

Preheat the oven to 220°C/425°F.

Wash the fish under cold running water and dry the inside and outside with paper towel. Trim the fins and tail with sharp scissors if your fishmonger hasn't done this for you. At 1cm/½in intervals, slash the flesh diagonally with a sharp knife.

Rub a third of the oil mixture and some salt (optional) inside each fish. Drizzle a third of the oil mixture over a large ovenproof serving dish or baking tray, sprinkle the surface with the scallions and place the fish on top.

Mix the lemon grass, ginger and garlic with the remaining oil, season with salt (optional) and pepper and spread the mixture all over the tops of the fish.

Cover the dish or baking tray with some kitchen foil and bake the fish in the oven for about 25 minutes or until the flesh is opaque. Remove the foil, sprinkle the fish with the cilantro and serve with Chinese-style steamed or stir-fried vegetables.

Spiced Mackerel

On a recent trip to the Isle of Wight, I returned loaded with freshly caught mackerel. I bought the gleaming fish already cleaned and beheaded so they just needed a quick wash and they were ready to be used in this quick and easy recipe.

If you can tolerate lactose, serve the fish with the raita accompaniment.

Serves 4

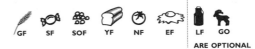

GF   SF   SOF   YF   NF   EF   LF   GO

ARE OPTIONAL

1 tablespoon organic coriander seeds

16 organic green cardamom pods, split and seeds scooped out

5cm/2in piece peeled organic root ginger, finely chopped

½ teaspoon organic ground cloves

Sea salt (optional) and freshly ground black pepper

4 tablespoons organic cold pressed extra virgin olive oil

4 fresh mackerel, cleaned, beheaded and washed under cold running water

2 tablespoons chopped fresh organic cilantro leaves

Raita

375ml/1½ cups natural organic goat's yogurt

1 large organic garlic clove, crushed

2 heaped tablespoons finely chopped fresh organic mint leaves

4 heaped tablespoons grated raw baby organic zucchini

In a large, non-stick skillet, heat the coriander and cardamom seeds for 2–3 minutes. Pound or process the hot spices with the ginger, cloves, salt (optional), pepper and oil in a pestle and mortar or food processor until you achieve a coating consistency.

Slash the skin of the fish diagonally on both sides and smear both sides with the spice mixture. Sauté the fish in large non-stick pan, over medium heat, until both sides are crispy and cooked through.

Meanwhile, make the raita by mixing the yogurt, garlic, mint and zucchini together in a small bowl.

Sprinkle the cooked mackerel with the cilantro and serve immediately, accompanied by the bowl of raita.

Asparagus Wrapped in Smoked Salmon with Dill Oil

This is the perfect quick but smart appetizer for a spring or summer dinner party. You can use salmon trout slices if you prefer and shredded basil leaves if you run out of fresh dill.

Serves 4

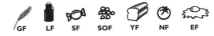

GF   LF   SF   SOF   YF   NF   EF

About 6 asparagus spears per person, trimmed of any tough stems

4 thick slices smoked wild salmon

A handful of prepared wild arugula

Organic cold pressed extra virgin olive oil for drizzling

Freshly ground black pepper

1 tablespoon finely chopped fresh organic dill

Cook the asparagus in boiling water until al dente, drain, rinse under cold running water and pat dry with kitchen paper.

When the asparagus is cold, divide into four bundles and wrap each bundle in a slice of thick smoked salmon. Place a bundle of asparagus on each plate and decorate with a few arugula leaves. In a small bowl, mix the oil with the pepper and dill, drizzle the mixture over the tips of the asparagus and serve immediately. You can keep them covered and chilled until needed but serve at room temperature.

Poultry and Game

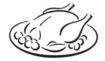

Chicken Liver Pâté

This simple and delicious pâté, which was such a hit in the 1970s, has now been revived and is once again popular as an appetizer or snack. Even though the usual sherry and cream ingredients have been omitted, this pâté is still creamy and rich.

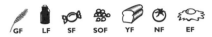

Serves 4

225g/8oz fresh or defrosted organic chicken livers, sinews or fat removed, rinsed under cold running water and drained

1 large organic onion, finely chopped (use a food processor)

2 tablespoons organic cold pressed extra virgin olive oil

85g/3oz/⅓ cup dairy-free vegetable margarine spread

Sea salt (optional) and freshly ground black pepper

Plenty of freshly grated nutmeg

2 heaped teaspoons each of fresh organic marjoram leaves, thyme leaves and chopped sage leaves

or 1 teaspoon each if using dried herbs

1–2 organic garlic cloves, chopped

Use clean fingers to separate the livers and leave to one side.

In a non-stick pan, gently cook the onion in the oil until softened but not browned. Stir in the livers and one-third of the margarine and cook until browned all over. Now add the salt (optional), pepper, nutmeg, herbs and chopped garlic. Shake the pan or stir from time to time until the livers are cooked through but just a tiny bit pink in the middle.

Remove the pan from the heat and leave the mixture to cool. Scrape the mixture into a food processor and blend until fairly smooth. Add the remaining margarine and blend again until smooth. Adjust the seasoning to taste and scrape the mixture into a serving dish. Cover and chill until needed.

Chicken Liver and Pine Nut Salad

Chicken livers are always much more tender and sweet if you take them off the heat when they are still just slightly pink. If you overcook them, they can be rubbery and dry. You can always cook them a fraction more if necessary but you can't reverse the effects of overcooking.

Serves 2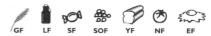

225g/8oz frozen organic chicken livers, defrosted, trimmed and divided into bite-size pieces

2 tablespoons organic cold pressed extra virgin olive oil

1 heaped teaspoon dried or fresh organic thyme leaves

1 heaped teaspoon dried or fresh chopped organic sage leaves

2 organic garlic cloves, crushed

Sea salt (optional) and freshly ground black pepper

40g/1½oz/¼ cup organic pine nuts

Plenty of freshly grated organic nutmeg

Enough organic salad for two — mixed organic leaves and herbs such as lettuce, arugula, baby spinach leaves, cilantro or basil leaves

Drizzle of Verjuice

Organic walnut oil for drizzling

Sauté the livers in the oil with the thyme, sage and garlic until browned but not quite cooked through. Season the livers with salt (optional) and pepper, stir in the pine nuts and nutmeg and cook for a few more minutes while you arrange the salad leaves on the plates.

Spoon the liver mixture onto the salads and serve immediately, drizzled with a little Verjuice and plenty of walnut oil.

Chicken, Fennel and Pine Nut Risotto

You can also make this risotto with organic turkey, salmon or shrimp. For a vegetarian version, you could use zucchini or fava beans.

Serves 4–5

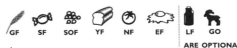

2 tablespoons organic cold pressed extra virgin olive oil

2 medium bulbs organic fennel, trimmed, tough outer layers removed, finely chopped

1 large organic onion, finely chopped

285g/10oz/1½ cups organic risotto rice

1 large organic garlic clove, crushed

1 liter/4 cups allergy-free vegetable bouillon

500g/1lb 2oz organic chicken breasts, trimmed and diced

55g/2oz/scant ½ cup organic pine nuts, toasted until golden

3 heaped tablespoons chopped fresh organic parsley

1 heaped tablespoon dairy-free vegetable margarine spread

Plenty of finely grated hard organic goat's cheese (optional)

Sea salt (optional) and freshly ground black pepper

Freshly grated organic nutmeg

Heat the oil in a non-stick pan over medium heat, add the fennel and onions and cook until softened. Stir in the rice and garlic; keep stirring for a minute or two and then add the bouillon. Bring the risotto to the boil and then simmer for about 15 minutes, stirring from time to time. If the liquid is absorbed too quickly you will have to add more water to prevent the rice from sticking to the pan.

Stir in the chicken, half the pine nuts and half the parsley and cook for about 20 minutes or until the rice and the chicken are cooked through and tender and the risotto is thick and creamy.

Stir the margarine and grated goat's cheese (if using) into the risotto and season according to taste with salt (optional), pepper and nutmeg. Serve hot, sprinkled with the remaining pine nuts and parsley.

Turkey Stroganoff

I have always made stroganoff with a variety of meats other than beef, and turkey is a good low-fat alternative. If you can't eat mushrooms then use another quick-cooking vegetable such as zucchini. Serve with steamed brown rice.

Serves 4

[contains mushrooms]
/GF   GO   SF   SOF   YF   NF   EF

4 tablespoons organic cold pressed extra virgin olive oil

1 large organic onion, halved and very finely sliced

455g/1lb organic turkey breast, cut into thin bite-size strips

2 heaped tablespoons organic rice flour

285g/10oz/3⅓ cups organic mushrooms, wiped clean and sliced

55g/2oz/¼ cup dairy-free vegetable margarine spread

250ml/1 cup strong organic chicken or turkey bouillon

Freshly grated organic nutmeg

Sea salt (optional) and freshly ground black pepper

2 heaped tablespoons chopped fresh organic parsley

2 heaped tablespoons double goat's cream or more according to taste

Heat half the oil in a non-stick skillet, add the onions and cook over gentle heat until they are nearly soft but not colored.

Turn the heat up and add the remaining oil to the pan. Now add the turkey, sprinkle with the flour and cook for a few minutes, over high heat, stirring the meat and onions. Reduce the heat to medium, add the mushrooms and margarine and cook for a few minutes. Add the bouillon and simmer until cooked through, stirring occasionally.

Sprinkle the stroganoff with the nutmeg, salt (optional), pepper and half the parsley. Stir in the cream, simmer the turkey for a few minutes and sprinkle with the remaining parsley.

Chicken with Almond and Coconut Sauce

The lovely mellow sauce in this recipe is also delicious spiced up with a bit of chili – but only if you can tolerate it of course. You can also make this dish using organic turkey or simply with your favorite vegetables.

Serves 4

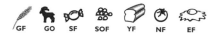

250ml/1 cup organic goat's yogurt

2 organic garlic cloves, crushed

5cm/2in piece organic fresh root ginger, peeled and grated

Plenty of coarsely ground black pepper and some sea salt (optional)

4 organic chicken breasts, trimmed and sliced into bite-size pieces

85g/3oz/⅓ cup dairy-free vegetable margarine spread

2 organic onions, halved and sliced

1 teaspoon each of the following: organic ground cumin, coriander seeds, cloves, cinnamon and
    turmeric

55g/2oz/½ cup ground organic almonds

200ml/¾ cup organic coconut cream

15g/½ oz/¼ cup fresh organic cilantro leaves, chopped

Mix the yogurt, garlic, ginger, pepper and salt (optional) in a bowl and stir in the sliced chicken. Cover and chill – preferably overnight; otherwise as long as possible.

Heat the margarine in a non-stick skillet over medium heat, add the onions and all the ground spices and cook gently until soft. Stir in the chicken and yogurt mixture and cook for a few minutes before adding the ground almonds and coconut cream. Simmer the chicken until tender, stirring from time to time, and serve sprinkled with the fresh cilantro leaves.

Stuffed Turkey Breasts and Saffron Sauce

Saffron usually comes in tiny amounts and although it is expensive you only need a few strands, so a pack will lasts for ages. Saffron is used in paella and other rice dishes, but don't keep it for too long as, like other spices, it will lose its pungency and aroma over time.

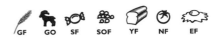

Serves 4

4 large thick organic turkey breast steaks, trimmed

400g/14oz/7 cups finely chopped frozen organic spinach

1 organic garlic clove, crushed

Sea salt (optional) and freshly ground black pepper

Freshly grated organic nutmeg

1 tablespoon organic cold pressed extra virgin olive oil

250ml/1 cup boiling allergy-free vegetable or chicken bouillon infused with a pinch

of saffron and left to cool

Finely chopped fresh cilantro leaves to serve

Sauce

1 tablespoon dairy-free vegetable margarine spread

1 tablespoon organic rice flour

125ml/½ cup organic goat's cream

Small wooden skewers or string

Place a turkey breast between two large pieces of wax paper and bash with a rolling pin or meat mallet to flatten the breast out into a large, thin escalope. Repeat with the remaining turkey breasts.

Gently cook the frozen spinach with the garlic, salt (optional), pepper and nutmeg in a non-stick pan until it is hot and the water has evaporated. Place a thick layer of paper towel on a plate and drain the spinach on it.

When the spinach is cold, spoon a quarter of the mixture in a line across the widest part of each turkey breast and then roll each one into a package. Secure with a little wooden skewer or tie up with string.

Sauté the turkey rolls in the oil, in a non-stick skillet, until lightly browned on all sides. Pour in the saffron bouillon, shake the pan over the heat and cook for a couple of minutes.

In a small bowl, beat the margarine with the flour until it resembles a paste then stir it into the pan. Stir and cook the sauce until it is smooth and thick. Stir in the goat's cream, salt (optional) and pepper and simmer until the juices run clear from the turkey when a skewer is inserted into the centre.

Transfer the turkey rolls and sauce onto a warm dish and serve immediately with a sprinkling of cilantro.

Pheasant with Fennel and Artichokes

I love the Mediterranean combination of fennel and artichokes. This dish is usually enhanced with the flavors of grated lemon rind and chili but here I have simply depended on garlic and herbs.

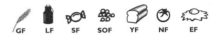

Serves 4–6

GF   LF   SF   SOF   YF   NF   EF

4–6 large plump oven-ready pheasant breasts, fat and skin removed

2 heaped tablespoons organic rice flour seasoned with freshly ground black pepper and sea salt (optional)

3 tablespoons organic cold pressed extra virgin olive oil

1 large organic onion, finely sliced

1 large organic fennel, trimmed of any tough layers and finely sliced

2 heaped teaspoons organic oregano leaves

2 organic garlic cloves, crushed

750ml/3 cups strong allergy-free chicken, pheasant or vegetable bouillon or consommé

395g/14oz can organic artichoke hearts, drained or use freshly cooked or frozen and defrosted

2 heaped tablespoons chopped fresh organic parsley

Preheat the oven to 190°C/375°F.

Dust the pheasant breasts with the seasoned flour. Heat the oil in a deep heat-proof casserole, add the pheasant breasts and sauté until golden. Now add the onions and cook over medium heat until the onions have softened. Add the fennel, oregano, garlic and bouillon, and stir. Cover and transfer to the oven.

Cook the casserole for about 55 minutes or until the pheasant is tender. Transfer the casserole to the stove-top and, over medium heat, stir in the artichokes and parsley. Adjust the seasoning and simmer for a few minutes until the artichokes have warmed through. Serve or cool and freeze.

Chicken, Bean Sprout and Water Chestnut Salad

This recipe is a combination of a stir-fry and salad – the chicken and flavourings make up the stir-fry while the bean sprouts and herbs give a crunchy salad effect.

Serves 2

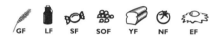

1 tablespoon organic sesame oil

2 tablespoons organic cold pressed extra virgin olive oil

2 organic chicken breasts, trimmed and sliced into bite-size pieces

225g/8oz can water chestnuts, drained

1 large organic garlic clove, crushed

1 tablespoon finely chopped lemon grass

5cm/2in piece organic root ginger, peeled and freshly grated

200g/7oz/2 cups organic bean sprouts

Freshly ground black pepper and sea salt (optional)

2 heaped tablespoons chopped fresh organic cilantro leaves

2 teaspoons organic sesame seeds

Heat the oils together in a wok, over high heat, for a few moments. Add the chicken and stir-fry it until sealed on all sides. Add the water chestnuts, garlic, lemon grass and ginger, stir and toss the mixture until the chicken is cooked through and tender. Remove the wok from the heat and stir in the bean sprouts, pepper, salt (optional) and the chopped cilantro leaves.

Serve the salad at room temperature, sprinkled with the sesame seeds.

Duck with Roast Asparagus and Thyme Jus

Duck has a wonderfully rich flavor that contrasts well with the clean taste of asparagus. Out of season, you can use batons of roast parsnip or sweet potato instead of asparagus.

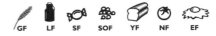

Serves 2

½ tablespoon organic rice flour

½ tablespoon dairy-free vegetable margarine

2 small organic duck breasts, skin and fat removed

A little organic cold pressed extra virgin olive oil

2 heaped teaspoons fresh organic thyme leaves

Freshly ground black pepper and sea salt (optional)

225g/8oz/1½ cup fresh organic asparagus, trimmed

125ml/½ cup strong allergy-free chicken or vegetable bouillon or consommé

Mix the rice flour and margarine together in a small bowl until smooth.

Brush the duck breasts with oil and sprinkle with thyme, pepper and salt (optional). Lightly score each duck breast, diagonally, using a sharp knife. Sauté the duck in a non-stick skillet, over medium heat, for about 3 minutes each side. Increase this cooking time for bigger duck breasts or if you don't like pink meat.

Meanwhile, cook the asparagus in boiling water for 3 minutes or until tender, then drain, arrange in a row on two warm plates and keep warm.

Add the bouillon to the pan and reduce for a few minutes, turning the duck over once.

Remove the duck from the pan and leave to one side for a couple of minutes while you thicken the thyme jus. Stir in the flour and margarine mixture and keep stirring over medium heat until the sauce is thick and glossy. Adjust the seasoning with salt (optional) and pepper and remove from the heat.

Carve the duck diagonally so that you have attractive-looking slices and arrange them over the asparagus. Pour over the thyme jus and serve immediately.

Venison Casserole with Cranberries and Spiced Pears

You can make double or triple the amount in this recipe and freeze the extra in containers for a later date. I tend to do this when venison is at its cheapest towards the end of the season.

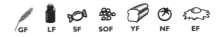

Serves 6

780g/1¾ lb venison meat, cut into bite-size cubes

2 heaped tablespoons organic rice flour seasoned with freshly ground black pepper and sea salt (optional)

4 tablespoons organic cold pressed extra virgin olive oil

2 large organic onions, very finely chopped

1 large organic carrot, peeled and very finely chopped

1 large stick organic celery, very finely chopped

1 small organic leek, tough outer leaves discarded, very finely chopped

(you can use the food processor for all the above chopping)

750ml/3 cups strong allergy-free chicken, game or vegetable bouillon or consommé

1 heaped teaspoon organic pie spice (check it is gluten-free)

3 organic bay leaves

2 heaped teaspoons organic marjoram leaves

225g/8 oz/2 cups fresh or frozen organic cranberries

2 large organic pears, just ripe enough to be able to quarter and core them but they must not be soft or bruised

2 heaped tablespoons chopped fresh organic parsley

Preheat the oven to 190°C/375°F.

Dust the venison in the seasoned flour. Heat the oil in a large heatproof casserole, add the venison and sauté over medium heat until browned all over.

Stir all the chopped vegetables into the casserole and brown for a few minutes, then stir in the bouillon or consommé and bring to boiling point. Remove the casserole from the heat and stir in the pie spice, bay leaves and marjoram. Cover and transfer to the oven to cook for 1 hour.

Remove the casserole from the oven and reduce the oven temperature to 150°C/300°F. Stir the cranberries and pears into the casserole, cover and return the casserole to the oven to cook for another hour.

Serve the venison casserole sprinkled with parsley.

This dish is delicious served with a purée of celeriac or parsnips. You can cool the venison casserole and chill for up to 24 hours. Reheat gently and serve sprinkled with freshly chopped parsley.

Turkey Escalopes in Herby Breadcrumbs

Without using eggs it is difficult to achieve a thick crust on the escalopes but by adding some lovely fresh herbs the overall effect is delicious.

Serves 4

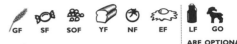

4 large thick organic turkey steaks, fat and skin removed

85g/3oz/1½ cups Orgran all-purpose allergy-free crumbs

1 teaspoon each finely chopped fresh organic rosemary and fresh organic thyme leaves

Sea salt (optional) and freshly ground black pepper

4 tablespoons organic cold pressed extra virgin olive oil

Optional

Finely sliced hard organic goat's cheese

Place each steak between 2 sheets of damp wax paper or plastic wrap and beat with a rolling pin or mallet until thin and evenly flattened. Mix the crumbs with the rosemary and thyme, and season with salt (optional) and pepper. Dip each escalope in a bowl of cold filtered water and then coat with as many crumbs as possible.

Heat half the oil in a non-stick skillet, add two escalopes at a time and sauté over medium heat for about 3 minutes on each side until golden, crispy and cooked through. Place the cooked escalopes on some thick paper towel and keep warm while you cook the remaining escalopes in the rest of the oil. Drain the last batch on more paper towel and serve immediately. Alternatively, place some thin slices of cheese on top of each escalope, broil until melted and serve immediately.

Meat

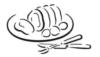

Lamb Kebabs

Kebabs are always popular and an easy option for a barbecue. Instead of the usual couscous salad to accompany the meat, I suggest you serve the kebabs with the Quinoa Risotto on page 196. Alternatively, serve a selection of salads and the Avocado and Mango Salsa on page 254.

Serves 4

[contains mushrooms] 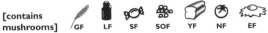 GF   LF   SF   SOF   YF   NF   EF

680g/1½ lb organic lamb, half leg or neck fillets trimmed and cut into 2.5cm/1in cubes

or use organic beef steaks

4 tablespoons organic cold pressed extra virgin olive oil

2 tablespoons Verjuice

2 teaspoons chopped fresh organic rosemary

Sea salt (optional) and freshly ground black pepper

1 large organic garlic clove, crushed

1 medium-sized organic red onion, peeled, quartered and separated into

12 thinner sections, blanched in boiling water for 5 minutes and then drained

12 organic chestnut mushrooms

2 small zucchini, cut into thick chunks, blanched in boiling water for

no more than 5 minutes and drained

Organic bay leaves

Marinate the lamb for 2 hours, or overnight, in the oil, Verjuice, rosemary, season-ing and garlic.

If you will be serving the kebabs with quinoa risotto, start making this 30 minutes before making the kebabs.

Remove the meat with a slotted spoon onto a plate and reserve the marinade.

Thread eight short or four long skewers alternately with lamb, onion, mushrooms, zucchini chunks and bay leaves.

Brush the kebabs with half the marinade, place on a baking tray a safe distance from the broiler and cook under high heat, turning once and basting again, until the meat is browned but still tender in the middle and the vegetables are tinged with brown.

Lamb Burgers with Avocado and Mango Salsa

Burgers have been around for a long time but combined with salsa they have a contemporary, more sophisticated appearance. The salsa recipe is also delicious served with broiled or barbecued lamb chops or steaks.

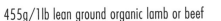

Serves 6

455g/1lb lean ground organic lamb or beef

½ organic red onion, minced

Sea salt (optional) and freshly ground black pepper

2 large organic garlic cloves, crushed

1 teaspoon dried or 2 of fresh organic thyme

Organic cold pressed extra virgin olive oil for brushing

Avocado and Mango Salsa (serves 6)

1 large ripe organic avocado, diced

½ organic red onion, diced

1 ripe organic mango, diced

Sea salt (optional) and freshly ground black pepper

6 tablespoons organic cold pressed extra virgin olive oil

4 tablespoons chopped organic basil or cilantro leaves

1 organic garlic clove, crushed

4 tablespoons Verjuice

Mix the lamb or beef with the minced onion, seasoning, garlic and thyme. Shape into burgers with clean hands and brush each one with a little oil.

Make the salsa: combine the diced avocado, onion and mango together in a bowl and mix in the seasoning, oil, herbs, garlic and Verjuice. Transfer the salsa to a serving bowl.

Broil the burgers on each side, under high heat, until cooked to your liking then serve immediately, with the salsa.

Carpaccio of Beef

Carpaccio of beef is usually cut wafer thin and served raw but here the beef is briefly cooked to give an interesting contrast in texture between the crust and the melt-in-the-mouth center. Beef fillet is ideal for eating cold so it makes an easy appetizer or main course.

Serves 4 as an appetizer

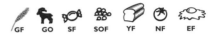

455g/1lb best organic beef fillet, from the tail end

Organic cold pressed extra virgin olive oil for brushing and drizzling

Sea salt (optional) and freshly ground black pepper

55g/2oz/1 cup prepared wild arugula

1 teaspoon truffle olive oil

1 teaspoon Verjuice

55g/2oz/½ cup hard organic goat's cheese

Make sure the meat is at room temperature. Heat a griddle pan over high heat until very hot and have a bowl of iced water ready. Brush the beef with a little of the oil and season with some salt (optional) and pepper.

Place the beef on the griddle and cook for 1 minute on each side and then another minute on each of the two edges (use tongs to do this). Quickly dip the sizzling meat in the iced water and pat dry with paper towel. Allow the meat to cool then refrigerate it until cold or cover and keep for up to 2 days.

Just before serving, toss the arugula in a bowl with a drizzle of olive oil, the truffle oil and a sprinkling of Verjuice. Arrange the leaves on four plates. Carve the beef into wafer thin slices and arrange over the leaves.

Use a potato peeler to shave curls of cheese over the top of each beef carpaccio, and serve.

Lamb Stir-fry with Snow Peas and Bok Choi

For a change from lamb, you could make this stir-fry with organic beef, chicken, turkey, duck or shrimp. Serve it with steamed fragrant Thai rice or basmati rice.

Serves 4

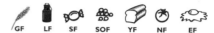

2 teaspoons organic sesame oil

2 tablespoons organic cold pressed extra virgin olive oil

625g/1lb 6oz trimmed and thinly sliced organic lamb cut from ½ leg fillet

1 large organic garlic clove, crushed

2 teaspoons Chinese or Thai ground spice (without chili if on a nightshade-free diet) or make up your own using equal parts of organic star anise, fennel seed, ground cinnamon, cloves, ginger and garlic powder

6–7 organic scallions, finely chopped

6 baby-sized organic bok choi, trimmed and halved

170g/6oz/2 cups organic snow peas, topped and tailed

2 tablespoons Furikake Japanese seasoning

2 tablespoons allergy-free lamb, chicken or vegetable bouillon

Plenty of freshly ground black pepper and a little sea salt (optional)

2–4 heaped tablespoons chopped fresh organic cilantro leaves

Heat the oils in a wok, add the lamb, garlic and spice mixture and sauté for a few minutes until the meat is browned all over. Add the scallions, bok choi and snow peas and stir-fry for a few minutes until softened. Stir in the Furikake seasoning, bouillon and seasoning to taste. Allow the mixture to bubble for a few minutes and serve immediately, sprinkled with the chopped cilantro leaves.

Steak and Black Peppercorns with Sweet Potato Fries

Steak and fries is such an easy treat and tastes extra special served with lots of delicious salad leaves, finely sliced vine tomatoes and fresh basil. The fries are also good served with broiled fresh fish or jumbo shrimp and garlic – or with roasted vegetables if you are a vegetarian.

GF   LF   SF   SOF   YF   NF   EF

Serves 2

Steaks

2 organic fillet, sirloin or rump steaks

1 tablespoon crushed black peppercorns

1 large organic garlic clove, crushed

1 tablespoon dairy-free vegetable margarine spread

Sea salt (optional)

1 tablespoon organic cold pressed extra virgin olive oil

Sweet potato chips

Cold pressed organic sunflower oil

2 small organic sweet potatoes, peeled and cut into slim fries

Roll the steaks in the black peppercorns. Beat the garlic and margarine together in a small cup and season with salt (optional).

Heat enough sunflower oil in a skillet, over medium heat, to sauté the sweet potatoes. Cook the fries in the oil until soft inside but golden and crispy on the outside. Drain them, transfer onto absorbent paper on a heatproof dish and keep them warm in a very hot oven.

Sauté the steaks in a skillet in the olive oil until cooked to your liking. About 1 minute before the end of the cooking time, add the garlic margarine and shake the pan until it has blended in with the steaks and juices.

Serve the steaks immediately with a pile of golden sweet potato fries.

Beef Casserole with Celeriac Croutons

In this casserole, I have used carrot juice and pumpkin purée instead of the usual combination of wine and tomato purée. It is still a rich and warming stew and is further enhanced by the subtlety of the celeriac.

Serves 6

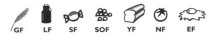

Casserole

1kg/2lb 4oz organic shin of beef, trimmed weight, chopped into cubes

4 heaped tablespoons organic rice flour seasoned with freshly ground black pepper and sea salt (optional)

3 tablespoons organic cold pressed extra virgin olive oil

250ml/1 cup organic carrot juice

500ml/2 cups strong allergy-free vegetable or beef bouillon

2 large organic onions, finely sliced

2 large organic carrots, chopped

3 organic bay leaves

2 teaspoons fresh or dried organic rosemary

2 large organic garlic cloves, crushed

2 tablespoons finely chopped fresh organic parsley to serve

Celeriac croutons

1 large organic celeriac, peeled, trimmed and cut into uniform bite-size cubes (use the offcuts and trimmings for soup or as flavoring for a mash)

1 teaspoon organic fresh or dried thyme leaves

Cold pressed organic sunflower oil

Preheat the oven to 180°C/350°F.

Toss the beef in the seasoned flour. Heat 2 tablespoons of the olive oil in a large heatproof casserole, add the beef and sauté until lightly browned. Stir in the carrot juice and bouillon and set aside. Sauté the onions in the remaining tablespoon of olive oil for a few minutes then stir them into the casserole. Add the carrots, herbs and garlic, cover and cook in the oven for about 1¼ hours or until the meat is tender.

Meanwhile, cook the celeriac in boiling water until softened but not cooked through. Drain the celeriac cubes and keep to one side until you are ready to sauté them. Remove the casserole from the oven but keep the lid on.

Sauté the celeriac cubes and thyme in some oil, over medium heat, until they are golden brown all over. Drain the croutons on absorbent paper towel.

Remove the lid from the casserole and stir the stew – it should be thick and glossy. Sprinkle the top with the croutons and parsley and serve immediately.

You can double the quantities and freeze the stew whole or in portions and make the celeriac croutons when the stew is reheated.

Braised Lamb with Flageolets and Thyme

Lamb shanks have been back in fashion for some time but it is essential that they are cooked long and slow so that the meat melts in the mouth. The dish can be frozen and reheated, which is ideal for easy entertaining. Serve with a purée of celeriac or parsnips.

Serves 4–8

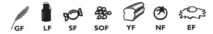

140g/5oz/¾ cup uncooked organic flageolets, soaked overnight, drained and boiled in fresh water until soft or according to the instructions on the packet or 2 x 300g/ 10½ oz cans unsweetened organic flageolets, drained and rinsed under cold running water

4 small leg shanks (you need the bone in to give the flavor)

2 tablespoons organic rice flour seasoned with freshly ground black pepper

3 tablespoons organic cold pressed extra virgin olive oil

2 teaspoons fresh or dried organic thyme

15g/½oz/½ cup fresh organic sage, trimmed

4 organic garlic cloves, crushed

4 organic bay leaves

2 large organic onions, halved and finely sliced

½ x 55g/2oz can anchovy fillets in olive oil, drained

250ml/1 cup allergy-free lamb, chicken or vegetable bouillon

250ml/1 cup organic carrot juice

Preheat the oven to 180°C/350°F.

First prepare the flageolets – the day before needed if they are dried.

Dust the lamb in the seasoned flour and then sauté in the oil in a large ovenproof casserole until browned all over. Add the thyme, sage, garlic, bay leaves and onions and cook for about 5 minutes over medium heat. Stir in the anchovy fillets, bouillon and carrot juice and bring to boiling point.

Cover the casserole and cook in the oven for about 1 hour. Remove the casserole from the oven, stir the ingredients so that they brown evenly and then mix in the prepared flageolets. Cover the casserole and return it to the oven to cook for 30 minutes or until the meat literally falls off the bone. Adjust the seasoning to taste and serve.

Desserts

Raspberry Frozen Yogurt

This recipe only takes about 30 minutes from start to finish, so as long as you have an ice cream maker you can whip up this dessert while you are eating your main course!

Do not freeze it and do not try to make half the quantity.

Serves 4

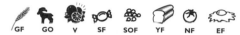

GF   GO   V   SF   SOF   YF   NF   EF

500g/17oz/2 cups plain unsweetened organic goat's yogurt
200g/7oz/1¾ cups very ripe fresh organic raspberries

Prepare and chill the ice cream maker for 5 minutes or as indicated by the manufacturer's instructions. Mix and stir the yogurt and raspberries together in a bowl and scrape into the chilled ice cream bowl. Churn until soft-frozen and serve immediately, either on its own or with a pile of ripe berries.

You should be able to make double the quantity in your ice cream maker.

Summer Fruit Terrine

Agar flakes are an excellent vegetarian alternative to gelatine and they can be used in mousses, gelatines and fools. If you want to make the terrine with fruits other than those specified, ensure that they are not too acidic or the dish won't set properly.

Serves 8

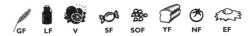

625ml/2½ cups organic unsweetened fruit juice (suitable for your diet) — I use peach and mango

2 rounded tablespoons agar flakes

500g/1lb 2oz/3½ cups fresh mixed organic summer berries (strawberries, raspberries, blueberries or pitted cherries), hulled and sliced or halved where necessary

Fresh organic mint to serve

900g/2lb loaf pan lined with plastic wrap, with a generous overhang

Pour the fruit juice into a small pan, sprinkle with the agar flakes and place over medium heat for about 3 minutes until dissolved – but do not stir.

Reduce the heat slightly and simmer the liquid, stirring from time to time, for about 2–3 minutes. Cool and leave for 10–15 minutes.

Fill the prepared loaf pan with the fruit. Stir the cooling liquid and pour it over the fruit. Leave the terrine to set in the refrigerator. Cover with plastic wrap once it has cooled and keep for up to 12 hours.

To serve, turn the terrine onto a serving plate and decorate with fresh mint. Serve in slices.

Plum Crumble

You can of course combine this crumble mixture with any sort of fruit that you fancy, preferably whatever is in season. I often freeze fruit mixtures in advance so that I can quickly put together a fresh crumble at the last minute.

Serves 6

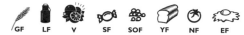

1kg/2lbs 4oz sweet organic eating plums, quartered and pitted or any other
prepared seasonal fruit, lightly stewed or poached in 125ml/½ cup filtered water

Crumble
55g/2oz/⅓ cup organic millet flour
135g/5½oz/1 cup organic rice flour
85g/3oz/⅔ cup ground organic almonds
1 teaspoon ground organic cinnamon
115g/4oz/½ cup dairy-free vegetable margarine spread
30g/1oz/⅓ cup unsweetened shredded organic coconut

Preheat the oven to 200°C/400°F.

Put the stewed or poached plums in an ovenproof serving dish and level off. Sprinkle with a little filtered water if there is very little juice.

Make the crumble by mixing the millet and rice flour, ground almonds, cinnamon, margarine and coconut together in a bowl. Rub the mixture lightly between your fingertips until you have fine crumbs and then spoon the crumble over the top of the plums. Gently pat the crumble with your hand so that the top is slightly firm.

Bake the crumble in the oven for about 30 minutes or until the fruit is bubbling and the crumble is golden brown.

Apricot and Almond Flan

This flan is glazed with arrowroot, a useful root starch because it has little taste and thickens small quantities of liquid. Arrowroot is refined from a West Indian plant (*Maranta arundinacea*) and can be found in supermarkets.

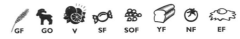

Serves 8

Pastry
30g/1oz/scant ¼ cup organic tapioca flour
30g/1oz/scant ¼ cup organic quinoa flour
170g/6oz/1¼ cups organic rice flour
70g/2½ oz/⅓ cup pure vegetable shortening
70g/2½ oz/⅓ cup dairy-free vegetable margarine spread
A pinch of fine salt (optional)
Cold filtered water

Filling
900g/2lbs/8 cups very ripe organic apricots, halved and pitted
4 tablespoons rose water
100–150g/3½–5oz/½–¾ cup soft organic goat's cheese
Pure vanilla extract to taste
About 125ml/½ cup organic goat's cream (according to the solidness of the cheese)
About 4 teaspoons arrowroot mixed with 250ml/1 cup unsweetened peach/apricot
or any other tolerated fruit juice mix
30g/1oz/⅓ cup flaked organic almonds, baked until golden brown

25.5cm/10in fluted non-stick tart pan lined with a circle of wax paper.

Preheat the oven to 190°C/375°F.

Make the pastry first. Using clean fingertips, mix and rub the flours, shortening, margarine and salt (optional) together in a bowl until the mixture resembles bread-crumbs. Then, using a blunt-edged knife to mix the dough, gradually add some filtered water, a little at a time, until it comes together in a ball. Alternatively, make the pastry in the food processor, giving it brief mixes at each stage.

Roll out the pastry on a floured board into a large enough circle to fit the base of your pan. Carefully lift the pastry into the pan, gently pushing out the pastry with your fingertips until it fits well. Prick the base with a fork and neaten the edges. Bake the pastry in the oven for about 20–25 minutes or until golden and slightly shrunk back from the pan. Leave to cool.

Meanwhile, put the apricots and rose water in a large non-stick pan and cover with a lid. Cook over low heat until the apricots are soft but have not begun to break up. Leave until cold.

Once the pastry base has cooled down, transfer it to a flat serving dish.

In a bowl, mix the soft goat's cheese with the vanilla and add the cream, a little at a time, until the mixture is smooth and spreadable but still thick. Cover the pastry with the cheese mixture, making sure that you go right to the edge all the way round. Cover with the apricots, starting from the outside and working inwards to the center. It doesn't matter if they are a bit squished up as you are going to glaze the fruit anyway.

Bring the arrowroot and fruit juice mixture to the boil in a small pan and stir until thick. Let the mixture cool a little and brush as much of the warm glaze over the apricots as you like before it sets. Sprinkle the almonds over the tart and chill until needed.

Coconut and Berry Fool

This is a firm favorite of mine as it's so easy and quick to make. Children and grown-ups alike enjoy this fool and it's particularly good served with a large bowl of fresh berries for extra vitamins, color and texture.

Serves 6

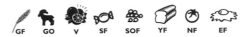

500g/1lb 2oz/3½ cups very ripe organic summer berries (in winter use frozen raspberries, blueberries, pitted cherries and strawberries, defrosted and drained of juices)

200ml/¾ cup chilled coconut cream

250ml/1 cup cold filtered water

2 rounded tablespoons agar flakes

250ml/1 cup chilled goat's cream

Optional

Extra berries for decoration

Purée the berries with the coconut cream in a blender and transfer to an attractive serving bowl. Combine the leftover juices, if there are any, with water so that you have 250ml/1 cup of liquid. Transfer to a small pan, sprinkle with the agar flakes and place over medium heat for about 3 minutes until dissolved – do not stir.

Reduce the heat slightly and simmer the liquid, stirring from time to time, for about 3 minutes. Set aside for 10–15 minutes until cool but not setting.

Quickly stir the mixture into the berry purée, wipe the sides of the bowl if necessary, cover and chill in the refrigerator until set.

Just before serving, decorate the top of the fool with a few extra berries. The fool is best eaten within 12 hours.

Baked Pear and Rice Pudding

You can use any non-acidic fruit in this recipe but make sure it isn't the kind that will produce lots of juice, or it will make the milk curdle. This recipe needs to be served warm, straight from the oven.

Serves 4

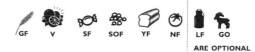

GF   V   SF   SOF   YF   NF   LF   GO

ARE OPTIONAL

3 heaped tablespoons organic pudding rice

A generous sprinkling of pure vanilla extract

2 ripe pears, peeled, halved, core discarded and then lightly poached or 425g/15oz can unsweetened organic pear halves, drained

625ml/2½ cups organic rice milk or goat's milk

15g/½ oz/1 tablespoon dairy-free vegetable margarine spread

Freshly grated organic nutmeg

Preheat the oven to 190°C/375°F

Sprinkle the rice over the bottom of an ovenproof serving dish about 20 x 24cm/8 x 10in in diameter. Sprinkle the vanilla over the rice and then arrange the pears over the top. Pour over the milk, dot with the margarine and dust with nutmeg.

Bake the rice pudding for about 1¼ hours or until the rice is tender and the pudding still milky. Serve immediately.

Strawberry and Blackberry Tart

I have found that a little tapioca flour is a very good and light substitute for wheat flour. Tapioca is derived from the root of a tropical plant known as manioc, or cassava, and is mainly used in puddings.

Serves 8

GF   GO   V   SF   SOF   YF   NF   EF

Pastry
30g/1oz/scant ¼ cup organic tapioca flour

30g/1oz/scant ¼ cup organic quinoa flour

170g/6oz/1¼ cups organic rice flour

70g/2½ oz/⅓ cup pure vegetable shortening

70g/2½ oz/⅓ cup dairy-free vegetable margarine spread

A pinch of fine salt (optional)

Cold filtered water

Filling
200g/7oz/1¾ cups fresh or frozen organic blackberries cooked with 125ml/½ cup filtered water or

1 x 290g/10oz can unsweetened blackberries, drained and liquid reserved

100–150g/3½ –5oz/½–¾ cups soft organic goat's cheese

Pure vanilla extract to taste

About 125ml/½ cup organic goat's cream (according to the solidness of the cheese)

450g/1lb/3 cups organic fresh strawberries, hulled then halved or quartered

About 4 teaspoons arrowroot mixed into the reserved cold blackberry juice (or 250ml/

1 cup of any other tolerated unsweetened red fruit juice)

22–23cm/8–9in fluted non-stick tart pan lined with a circle of wax paper

Preheat the oven to 190°C/375°F.

Make the pastry first. Using clean fingertips, mix and rub the flours, shortening, margarine and salt (optional) together in a bowl until the mixture resembles bread-crumbs. Then, using a blunt-edged knife to mix the dough, add some filtered water, a little at a time, until it comes together in a ball. Alternatively, make the pastry in a food processor, giving it brief mixes at each stage.

Roll out the pastry on a floured board into a large enough circle to cover the base and come some of the way up the sides of your dish. Using the rolling pin to help you, carefully lift the pastry into the pan, gently mold and push it out with your clean fingertips until it fits. Prick the base with a fork and neaten the edges. Bake the pastry in the oven for about 20–25 minutes or until golden and slightly shrunk back from the pan.

Meanwhile, if you are using fresh blackberries, place them in a non-stick pan, cover with a lid and cook over low heat until the fruit is softened and juicy. Remove the fruit from the heat before it begins to break up and leave until cold.

Let the pastry base cool down before transferring it to a flat serving dish.

In a bowl, mix the soft goat's cheese with the vanilla and add the cream, a little at a time, until smooth and spreadable. Cover the pastry with the cheese mixture, making sure that you go right to the edge all the way round. Cover with the straw-berries, starting from the outside and working inwards to the center. Use the black-berries to cover up any gaps but make sure the fruit looks nice.

Bring the arrowroot and fruit juice mixture to the boil in a small pan and stir until thick. Allow it to cool a little and brush as much of the warm glaze over the berries as you like. Serve at room temperature or chill until needed.

Rose-scented Peaches with Raspberry Sauce

Fresh peaches are my favorite summer fruit but I can never quite decide whether I prefer delicate white peaches or lush golden peaches. As I firmly believe that fruit should be eaten in its natural season, this pudding is the perfect combination.

Serves 4–6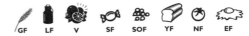

GF   LF   V   SF   SOF   YF   NF   EF

4–6 ripe organic peaches, peeled, halved and stones discarded

1 tablespoon rose water mixed with 5 tablespoons of just-boiled filtered water

170g/5oz/1cup very ripe hulled fresh organic raspberries or more if you prefer a really thick sauce

Optional

Some lightly toasted flaked organic almonds and/or 4–6 tiny sprigs of fresh organic mint

Place the peach halves in a shallow dish, cavity-side down, pour over the hot rose water and leave for about 10 minutes.

Carefully place 2 peach halves, cavity-side up, in each serving dish. Pour the rose water into a blender and blend with the raspberries until smooth. Sieve the purée into a bowl, discard the pips and spoon the sauce over the peaches.

Serve the peaches at room temperature, decorated with flaked almonds or fresh mint.

Breakfast and Afternoon Treats

In-the-Pink Smoothie

Smoothies provide a quick fix of fruit and yogurt and are a simple way of boosting your daily fruit quota. If the fruit featured is out of season, use high-quality frozen fruit – it's still packed with vitamins and it's convenient.

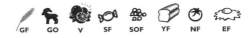

GF   GO   V   SF   SOF   YF   NF   EF

Serves 1–2

100g/3½ oz/1⅓ cups ripe organic blueberries

100g/3½ oz/1¼ cups ripe organic raspberries

1 large ripe organic banana, sliced

2 heaped tablespoons plain unsweetened organic goat's yogurt

250ml/1 cup organic goat's milk

Place all the ingredients in a food blender and blend until smooth. Pour the smoothie into two glasses and serve immediately.

Feeling Fruity Granola

Granola is a good sustaining start to the day, particularly when served with your allergy-free milk or unsweetened fruit juice and topped with goat's yogurt and seeds.

GF   V   SF   SOF   YF   NF   EF | LF   GO

ARE OPTIONAL

Basic mix

100g/3½oz/½ cup organic quinoa

100g/3½oz/½ cup organic amaranth

200g/7oz/2 scant cups organic rice flakes

100g/3½oz/1 scant cup organic millet flakes

55g/1oz/scant ½ cup chopped organic hazelnuts

55g/1oz/scant ½ cup chopped organic walnuts

100g/3½oz/½ cup organic dried apricots, chopped

100g/3½oz/½ cup organic dried figs, chopped

A good pinch organic ground cinnamon and grated nutmeg

Topping

Fresh organic berries

Plain unsweetened organic goat's yogurt (optional)

Organic sesame seeds

Mix the cereals together in a bowl. Broil the nuts on a baking tray until golden and mix into the bowl of cereals. Stir in the dried fruits and spices, transfer to a container, seal and store until needed.

The granola is even better if you leave it to soak for 10–30 minutes in your choice of milk or juice. Top with the berries, the yogurt, if using, and the seeds.

Fruity Spice Cake

I find this cake very useful for providing a fruity boost in lunch boxes or for picnics, as it travels well when sliced and wrapped in foil. It's also very popular as a mid-afternoon or after-school treat.

Serves 10
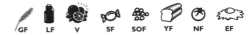

250g/9oz/2 cups pitted organic dates, chopped into small pieces

300ml/1¼ cups filtered water

85g/3oz/⅔ cup organic rice flour

85g/3oz/½ cup organic tapioca flour

3 teaspoons gluten-free baking powder

1 teaspoon ground organic cinnamon

1 teaspoon ground organic allspice

500g/1lb 2oz/3½ cups mixed dried organic fruits – raisins, currants, golden raisins

55g/1oz/½ cup ground organic almonds

80ml/⅓ cup organic pear, peach or apricot juice (or any suitable combination you enjoy)

900g/2lb loaf tin (pan) lined with non-stick wax paper

Preheat the oven to 180°C/350°F.

Put the dates in a small pan with the water. Bring to the boil, cook for a couple of minutes and remove from the heat. Sieve the flours, baking powder and spices into a bowl and mix in the dried fruit and almonds. Stir in the date mixture and the fruit juice and spoon the mixture into the prepared pan.

Bake for about 45 minutes or until a skewer, inserted into the middle of the cake, comes out clean. Cool the cake in the pan, then transfer to a wire rack and remove the wax paper. Serve the cake in slices.

Ginger and Apricot Loaf

I find this cake very popular with all age groups – it can be sliced and wrapped in foil for a child's lunch box, it's a great hit at picnics and is delicious served simply with a cup of herbal tea.

Serves 10

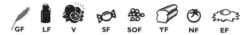

250g/9oz/2 cups pitted organic dates, chopped into small pieces

300ml/1¼ cups filtered water

85g/3oz/⅔ cup organic rice flour

85g/3oz/½ cup organic tapioca flour

3 teaspoons gluten-free baking powder

2 teaspoons organic ground ginger

1 teaspoon organic ground mixed spice (check label for gluten or make your own)

500g/1lb 2oz/3½ cups dried organic apricots, chopped into small pieces

55g/2oz/½ cup organic ground almonds

80ml/⅓ cup organic prune, peach or apricot juice (or any suitable combination you enjoy)

900g/2lb loaf pan lined with non-stick wax paper

Preheat the oven to 180°C/350°F.

Put the dates in a small pan with the water. Bring to the boil, cook for a couple of minutes and remove from the heat. Sieve the flours, baking powder and spices into a bowl and mix in the apricots and almonds. Stir in the wet date mixture and the fruit juice and spoon the mixture into the prepared pan.

Bake for about 45 minutes or until a skewer inserted into the middle comes out clean.

Leave the cake to cool in the pan, then transfer to a wire rack and remove the wax paper. Serve the cake in slices.

Banana and Walnut Muffins

While these delicious muffins bake, why not whiz up a smoothie or enjoy a bowl of fruity granola (see page 277) with fresh berries? I can't think of a better way to set yourself up for the day.

Makes 8

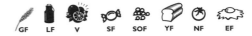

2 medium-sized ripe organic bananas

55g/2oz/generous ⅓ cup organic sultanas (golden raisins)

55g/2oz/generous ⅓ cup chopped organic dates

55g/2oz/generous ½ cup chopped organic walnuts

1 teaspoon organic ground cinnamon

1 teaspoon ground mixed spice (check it is gluten-free)

225g/8oz/1½ cups organic rice flour

1 teaspoon gluten-free baking powder

1 teaspoon baking soda

1 teaspoon cream of tartar

1 teaspoon vitamin C powder

1 tablespoon organic walnut oil

250ml/1¼ cups sugar-free prune juice

1 non-stick muffin pan, lined with 8 circles of non-stick wax paper
Preheat the oven to 200°C/400°F.

Coarsely mash the bananas and place in a bowl with the dried fruit, nuts and spices. Briefly stir all the remaining ingredients into the mixture. Spoon the muffin mixture into the prepared pan and bake for about 15–20 minutes or until firm to touch.

Cool the muffins in the pan, transfer to a wire rack, remove the wax paper and serve warm.

Appendices

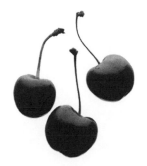

How to Do a Pulse Test

A pulse test is one of the best ways of finding out what foods you have an intolerance to. It is not too complicated – this appendix includes full instructions along with a brief history of the test.

In the text that follows the words 'allergy' or 'allergenic' will be used, but refer in this case to intolerance.

A Brief History of Pulse Testing

In the 1950s, Dr. Arthur Coca identified that his wife's heart rate would increase if she ate a food that provoked an inappropriate or allergic response. This was, as Dr Coca put it, 'accidentally acquired knowledge' which he then applied to patients as well as his wife. The results were very effective and consistent – in his wife's case, all symptoms disappeared.

Dr. Coca had to rely on observation, given the relative lack of sophisticated blood tests that are more available today. He developed a rational approach to measuring the pulse and its connection with foods, and used the technique to help many thousands of people. He also identified a number of symptoms:

Recurrent headache	Abnormal tiredness
Nervousness	Indigestion (vomiting, gas, nausea)
Migraine	Neuralgia
Dizziness	Sinusitis
Constipation	Hypertension
Heartburn	Hives
Canker sores	Angina
Epilepsy	Asthma
Overweight	Hemorrhoids
Underweight	Depression
Gastric ulcer	Diabetes
Abdominal pain	Chest pain
Gallbladder pain	Gastro-intestinal bleeding
Nervousness and emotional instability	Nose bleed
Colitis	

By applying the pulse test, as described below, Dr. Coca was able to resolve the above conditions in patients – but he also observed some corroborating evidence:

1. Patients usually had more than one of the above symptoms, all of which resolved when they avoided foods which made their pulse accelerate.
2. Symptoms were triggered by consuming the offending foods
3. When the offending foods were eaten there was a speeding up of the heart rate each and every time.

Given the impressive simplicity of the pulse test, I am going to describe how you can do it for yourself. You may feel that undertaking the test is a little beyond your capacity, but having done the testing myself I can tell you that it is actually quite fun and makes for a powerful way of proving your reactions. Dr. Coca called it a 'special medical diagnostic art'.

HOW TO DO THE PULSE TEST

1. Stop smoking entirely, as this will interfere with the pulse testing.
2. The pulse can be taken wherever it can be felt – in the wrist, at the neck or at the temple.
3. Count the number of beats for a whole minute, not less (e.g. do not count for 30 seconds and then double it).
4. Prepare a piece of paper on which to record your results. It should look something like the one below (page 288).
5. Count your pulse before and after each meal, as follows: just before eating the meal, then 30 minutes after the meal, 60 minutes after the meal and 90 minutes after the meal. Also take your pulse at bedtime, sitting on the bed.
6. All pulse counts are to be made while sitting down, except the first one of the day when you should be lying in bed.
7. Record everything eaten at each meal.
8. Continue to do this for two to three days with the usual three meals.
9. This means you should take your pulse 14 times a day (if you eat 3 meals).

Date:

Before rising (i.e. while still lying down)   pulse   xx

30 minutes after breakfast   xx

60 minutes after breakfast   xx

90 minutes after breakfast   xx

Foods eaten

....

....

....

Before lunch   pulse   xx

30 minutes later   xx

60 minutes later   xx

90 minutes later   xx

Foods eaten

....

....

....

Before Dinner   pulse   xx

30 minutes later   xx

60 minutes later   xx

90 minutes later   xx

Foods eaten

....

....

....

Bedtime Pulse   xx

If the pulse increases after a meal, it is then possible to determine which foods might be the offending items.

1. Take your before-rising pulse count as usual. This number will be your benchmark against other pulse counts throughout the day. However, if the count is lower later on in the day, then note this new low level and revise your benchmark rate accordingly.

2. Work out your highest normal maximum pulse rate during the day, when you are at rest. The difference between your lowest and highest pulse rate should be no more than 16 beats per minute. If the difference is greater, it suggests that there is some kind of allergy present.

3. Taking your lowest pulse rate as the benchmark, add 12 beats to give you an idea of the probable threshold above which there is likely to be some kind of allergic response, be it to a food or to something you have inhaled.

4. The next stage of testing is to isolate each food to determine which one is causing a problem. This is called single-food testing, which also needs to be done over two or three days. This involves snacking on single foods throughout the day.

5. Eat a small portion of a different food every hour. For example, a piece of bread, an egg, a piece of fruit. Take your pulse just before eating the food and 30 minutes afterwards. Do not test any food that you know disagrees with you.

Interpreting Your Pulse Record

If your pulse goes up noticeably after rising, it usually means you have a reaction to something like your toothpaste or toilet articles such as shaving lotion or make-up. Sometimes it can be newsprint off the morning paper.

There are also some basic rules that you can apply, although there may be exceptions to the rule:

1. If ingesting a frequently-eaten food causes no acceleration of your pulse (at least 6 beats above your normal maximum), that food can be tentatively considered non-allergenic for you. If ingesting it does cause acceleration of your pulse (30, 60, or 90 minutes after eating the food), it is likely you are allergic/sensitive to it and shouldn't eat it.

2. If you take your pulse at least 14 times a day, and if your daily maximum pulse-rate is constant (within one or two beats) for three days in succession, this indicates that all food-allergens have been avoided on those days.

3. If your daily maximum pulse-rate varies by more than two beats – for example, Monday 72, Tuesday 78, Wednesday 76, Thursday 71 – you are certainly allergic, provided there is no infection.

4. Pulse rates that are not more than 6 beats above the normal daily maximum should not be blamed on a recently eaten food, but on an inhalant or a recurring reaction.

5. If your minimum pulse rate does not regularly occur before rising, after the night's rest, but at some other time in the day, this usually indicates sensitivity to the house-dust mites found in mattresses or pillows.

6. If your pulse-count taken standing is greater than that taken sitting, this is a positive indication of present allergic tension.

Dr. Coca emphasized the importance of applying yourself to testing over a number of days in order to identify which foods are making your pulse faster than normal. Dr. Coca maintained that the method was a 'roadmap to the fountain of youth' and encouraged everyone to use it.

Appendix II

Food Intolerance Lab Tests
and Where to Get Them

There is no single food intolerance test that will identify every food to which you have an intolerance or negative reaction, but they can be of tremendous value in assessing those foods you should avoid or strictly limit.

In order to gain access to a very reliable and accurate test for food intolerances, I recommend you contact Immuno Laboratories in Florida, which has been involved in this field since 1978.

Immuno Laboratories, Inc.
6801 Powerline Road
Fort Lauderdale
Florida 33309
Tel: 954-691-2500
Toll-free: 1-800-231-9197
Fax: 954-691-2505
email: CSTWebmail@betterhealthusa.com
website: www.ImmunoLabs.com

To order a specimen kit, you will need to speak to a consultant. When you call ImmunoLabs' main number (800-231-9197) and ask for a specimen kit, the receptionist will connect you to the consultant that covers your area. That consultant will then help you with the process for obtaining specimen kits.

Food Intolerance Tests

- Standard Panel (115 foods)
- Pediatric Panel (88 Foods)
- Kosher Panel (108 Foods)
- Vegetarian Panel (104 Foods)

There is a 72-hour turnaround for the results.

Foods Tested for Each of the Panels

Standard Panel (115 Foods)

alfalfa	bean (pinto)	cashew nut	coconut
almond	bean (yellow wax)	cauliflower	cod
amaranth	beef	celery	coffee
apple	beet	cheese	corn
asparagus	brazil nut	cherry	crab
avocado	broccoli	chicken	cranberry
banana	Brussels sprouts	chili pepper	egg
barley	buckwheat	cinnamon	eggplant
bean (green)	cabbage	clam	flounder
bean (kidney)	Cantaloupe	clove	garlic
bean (lima)	carrot	cocoa/chocolate	ginger

grape	nutmeg	pork	spinach
grapefruit	oat	potato, sweet	strawberry
haddock	olive	potato, white	sugar, cane
halibut	onion	pumpkin	sunflower
herring	orange	quinoa	tangerine
lamb	oregano	radish	tea
lemon	oyster	rape seed (Canola)	tomato
lentil	papaya	rice	trout
lettuce	parsley	rye	tuna
lime	pea	safflower	turkey
lobster	peach	sage	walnut
mackerel	peanut	salmon	wheat
milk (cow's)	pecan	scallops	whitefish
milk (goat's)	pepper, black/white	sesame	yam
millet	pepper, green	shrimp	yeast, baker's
mung bean	perch	snapper	yeast, brewer's
mushroom	pineapple	sole	zucchini
mustard	plum	soybean	

Pediatric Panel (88 Foods)

Standard Panel with the following foods eliminated:

alfalfa, asparagus, chili pepper, clam, coffee, eggplant, flounder, garlic, haddock, halibut, herring, lobster, mackerel, mushroom, mustard, onion, oyster, parsley, perch, radish, salmon, scallops, shrimp, snapper, sole, trout, whitefish

Kosher Panel (108 Foods)

Standard Panel with the following foods eliminated:

clam, crab, lobster, oyster, pork, scallops, shrimp

Vegetarian Panel (104 Foods)

Standard Panel with the following foods eliminated:

beef, chicken, clam, crab, lamb, lobster, oyster, pork, scallops, shrimp, turkey

Appendix III

Other Lab Tests Available

Here are the details of the tests, other than the food intolerance tests or the pulse test, that may have been indicated by your scores in the questionnaires or that you simply wish to do because you believe they may show some important information of relevance to your health. The costs below are current at the time of publication and may fluctuate.

Test Name	Available from	Retail Cost	No. of Days
Adrenocortex Stress Profile (saliva)	Genova Diagnostics		7
Yeast Culture (stool)	Doctor's Data	$44.00	5-7
Comprehensive Stool Analysis (stool)	Doctor's Data	$331.00	5-7
Comprehensive Stool Analysis with Parasitology x1 (stool)	Doctor's Data	$397.00	5-7
Comprehensive Parasitology x1 (stool)	Doctor's Data	$159.00	5-7
Helicobacter Pylori Antigen (stool)	Doctor's Data	$99.00	3-5
Intestinal Permeability (urine)	Doctor's Data	$77.00	3-5
Hepatic Detox Profile (urine)	Doctor's Data	$218.00	3-5
Secretory IgA (SIgA) (stool)	Doctor's Data	$44.00	3-5

Doctor's Data, Inc.

3755 Illinois Avenue

St Charles

Illinois 60174-2420

Tel: 800-323-2784 or 630-377-8139

Fax: 630-587-7860

email: inquiries@doctorsdata.com

website: www.doctorsdata.com

Genova Diagnostics

63 Zillicoa Street

Asheville

North Carolina 28801

Tel: 800-522-4762

Fax: 828-252-9303

website: https://www.gdx.net/secure/contact/

When contacting either of these two laboratories, it is important to let them know you are a reader of this book and wish to undertake one of their tests. The labs will then refer you to a practitioner closest to you who will facilitate the tests for you.

Adrenocortex Stress Profile (saliva)

This is a saliva test, taking 4 samples at specific times during the day which are then sent off by mail directly to Genova Diagnostics. Saliva samples can be easily collected by the patient at home or at work. The Adrenocortex Stress Profile accurately measures unbound levels of both cortisol and DHEA, and provides a complete circadian analysis of cortisol activity. Controlled collection times allow for accurate baseline testing and effective monitoring of hormone replacement therapy.

Results take approximately 7 working days.

Relevance

The levels of stress hormones in your body have a profound effect on both gut immunity, including SIgA levels, and the ability of your body to heal your gut lining. This is also an indicator of how stress might be directly influencing your digestive function, as well as how much your digestive symptoms may have taxed your adrenals via the hypothalamus and pituitary. This profile serves as a critical tool for uncovering biochemical imbalances that can underlie anxiety, chronic fatigue, obesity, diabetes and a host of other clinical conditions. Since it is not always possible to determine from symptoms what your cortisol and DHEA levels are, the test is vital if you want to be able to target remedial help. If the test is not done, then it is suggested that you consider the general Adrenal Support Program.

Yeast Culture (stool)

This is a stool test that is sent by mail to the lab for analysis.

Results take approximately 7 working days.

Relevance

Infection with yeast species can cause a variety of symptoms, both within and outside the digestive system, and may escape suspicion as a pathogenic agent in many cases. Episodes of yeast infection after short-term and long-term antibiotic use have been identified in patients with both gastrointestinal and vaginal symptoms.

There is some evidence linking yeast infections with more chronic conditions outside the digestive tract. Studies suggest that the production of antibodies against *Candida albicans* may contribute to atopic dermatitis in young adults. Other studies have identified the potential role of candidiasis in chronic fatigue syndrome.

Identification of abnormal levels of specific yeast species in the stool is an important diagnostic step in therapeutic planning for the patient with chronic gastrointestinal and extra-gastrointestinal symptoms.

Yeast sensitivities to a variety of prescriptive and natural agents are provided when yeast is cultured at any level. This provides the clinician with useful information to help plan an appropriate treatment protocol.

Comprehensive Stool Analysis (stool)

This stool test involves samples from separate days that are sent off in special containers in the post directly to Doctor's Data. The results of the stool analysis tells you about a number of different aspects of digestive function, including markers of digestion such as pancreatic enzyme levels, markers of absorption, markers of inflammation, levels of friendly bacteria, levels of unwanted bacteria, levels of yeast, and presence of parasites.

Results take approximately 7 working days.

Relevance

If you have something wrong with your digestion or an imbalance in your bacteria levels (dysbiosis) then not only can this be a cause of food intolerances but it can be more difficult to resolve them. This test gives insight into what digestive imbalances you need to redress, which may vary from the need for digestive enzymes to the need for an anti-bacterial agent or use of a probiotic. The test analyzes for markers of digestion and inflammation as well as bacteria (good and bad) and yeasts. For those of you with digestive complaints this test could prove as valuable as a food intolerance test. There are various programs to follow should the tests yield positive results (i.e. something wrong): the Digestive Support Program, the Anti-Yeast Program, the Anti-Bacterial Program, and the Probiotic Support Program. This test does NOT analyze for parasites, which makes it of limited use since it excludes those with a score of 10 or more in the questionnaire 'Have I got parasites?' (page 75).

Comprehensive Stool Analysis with Parasitology x1 (stool)

This stool test involves samples from separate days that are sent off in special containers by mail directly to Doctor's Data. The results of the stool analysis tell you about a number of different aspects of digestive function, including markers of digestion such as pancreatic enzyme levels, markers of absorption, markers of inflammation, levels of friendly bacteria, levels of unwanted bacteria, levels of yeast, and presence of parasites.

Results take approximately 7 working days.

Relevance

If you have something wrong with your digestion or you have a yeast overgrowth or parasites, then not only can this be a cause of food intolerances, but it can be extremely difficult to resolve them. This test gives insight into what imbalances you need to redress, which may vary from an anti-parasitic program to a course of probiotics with digestive enzymes. For those of you with digestive complaints this test could prove as valuable as a food intolerance test. There are various programs to follow should the test yield positive results (i.e. something wrong): the Digestive Support Program, the Anti-Yeast Program, the Anti-Bacterial Program, the Anti-Parasitic Program, and the Probiotic Support Program.

Comprehensive Parasitology x1 (stool)

This stool test is simply assessing for yeast, bacteria and parasites, and not for other markers of digestion. It also involves two samples on two separate days that are sent off in special containers by mail directly to Doctor's Data. The results of the stool analysis tell you whether you are 'bugged' or not, and also provides you with an idea about how to address the unwelcome guests should there be any. This test is half the price of the Comprehensive Digestive Stool Analysis with Parasitology and should be considered instead of the previously mentioned test if there are strong indications that your health problems are very much related to 'bugs' as opposed to maldigestion. Check your scores for the questionnaires 'Have I got a yeast overgrowth?' and 'Have I got parasites?' to determine the basis for your need for this test.

Results take approximately 7 working days.

Relevance

Parasites and other unwelcome guests are a potential cause of food intolerance. There are various programs to follow should the test yield positive results (i.e. something wrong): the Anti-Yeast Program, the Anti-Bacterial Program, the Anti-Parasitic Program, and the Probiotic Support Program.

Helicobacter Pylori Antigen (stool)

While a blood test is available which measures antibody levels to *Helicobacter pylori*, this will only identify individuals who have been exposed to the bacterium at some time in their lives. It does not distinguish if there is a current infection. Since the antibodies to *H. Pylori* take some time to diminish, it is not a useful test by which to monitor treatment, whereas the stool test is.

The simple stool antigen test is able to confirm that there is an active current infection of *H. pylori*. The test involves providing a stool sample in the kit provided and mailing directly to Doctor's Data.

Results take approximately 5 working days.

Relevance

This is a relevant test if you have already been shown to have low stomach acid or symptoms of excess acid, and you need to rule out the presence of this bacterium. Low stomach acid is a potential root cause for maldigestion, unwanted gastro-intestinal bugs and consequently food intolerances.

Interpreting your results

Doctor's Data will help direct you to a practitioner who can help to interpret your results.

Intestinal Permeability (urine)

This is a test which involves collecting urine after drinking a special solution that helps to identify the size of molecules that gets through the gut lining and ends up in the urine.

Results take approximately 5 working days.

Relevance

You can assume that you have a leaky gut if you have food intolerances, and therefore this has little relevance UNLESS you have very few digestive complaints (Section One of the Food Intolerance Questionnaire) and score more highly on mental, emotional and nervous system symptoms (Section Two of the Food Intolerance Questionnaire). This test is therefore recommended if your major complaints are nervous system-related, since it will be important both to avoid culprit foods and to look to heal the gut lining with specific remedies, as described in the Gut Healing Program.

Hepatic Detox Profile (urine)

Three compounds, caffeine, acetaminophen, and acetylsalicylic acid, are taken orally to challenge the liver's Phase I and Phase II detoxification capacity. They are sent directly to Doctor's Data where the saliva and urine are analyzed for metabolites of the three compounds to determine how well the liver can convert and clear toxins from the body. This test is NOT recommended for children 12 years old and younger.

Results take approximately 5 working days.

Relevance

This test is not a typical front-line test from the perspective of those suffering from food intolerances, unless there are very few digestive symptoms. It is usually most important to address the digestive problems as a priority. However, it is almost always a second line test to consider since the liver has to deal with all matter that gets absorbed through your gut lining. Protocols are provided for general liver support and if your Phase I enzymes are imbalanced either way with Phase II enzymes.

Secretory IgA (SIgA) (stool)

This involves providing a single stool sample and sending it by mail directly to Doctor's Data. The results show your level of SIgA within a reference range.

Results take approximately 5 working days.

Relevance

SIgA is the most abundant immunoglobulin your body produces and it coats your gut lining and mucus membranes as a defensive barrier. A number of factors such as stress and gut infections (yeast, bacterial or parasitic) can deplete your SIgA which then increases the risk of food intolerances and infection by unwelcome visitors. It can be more difficult, if not impossible, to resolve food intolerances in the long term unless SIgA levels are optimized. This is one of the tests you should do if you make no evident progress in four weeks on the approaches described in this book, which should ordinarily support SIgA levels themselves but not as specifically as the SIgA Support Program. The Adrenocortex Stress Profile test also has strong relevance to the SIgA result.

Appendix IV

Supplement Information
and Websites

This appendix tells you how to order the nutritional supplements in this book and summarizes the remedial plans described in Chapter 7.

You can obtain all of the supplements referred to in this book from the Allergy Research Group and the Biotics Research Corporation, by contacting the two companies directly.

Allergy Research Group

2300 North Loop Road

Alameda

California 94502

Tel: 800-545-9960 or 510-263-200

Fax: 800-688-7426 or 510 263-2100

email: info@allergyresearchgroup.com

website: www.allergyresearchgroup.com

Biotics Research Corporation

6801 Biotics Research Drive

Rosenberg

Texas 77471

Tel: 800-231-5777 or 281-344-0909

Fax: 281-344-0725

website: www.BioticsResearch.com

When you contact these companies they will do their best to direct you to a practitioner as close to you as possible who is familiar with the use of these products, so that you can purchase them directly or gain further assistance from them.

Summary of the Remedial Programs detailed in this book

Supplement Plans

- Digestive Support Plan
- Digestive Support Plan 2
- Digestive Support Plan 3
- Anti-*Helicobacter Pylori* Plan
- Gut Lining Support Plan
- Anti-Yeast Plan
- Anti-Parasitic Plan
- SIgA Plan
- Adrenal Support Plan
- General Liver Support Plan
- Liver Support Plan – Higher Phase I than II
- Liver Support Plan – Lower Phase I than II

Adrenal Protocols for results of the Adrenocortex Stress Profile (saliva) are available on request. There are currently 25 of them, and it is not possible to display all of these on the website. Simply email me on antonyjhaynes@aol.com, letting me know your test results (i.e. your cortisol and DHEA) results and I will send you the appropriate protocol that suits your result.

Appendix V

Foods Containing Salicylate

This book does not cater specifically to those with a salicylate sensitivity, and the challenge of excluding this component of food as well as all the 'Usual Suspects' would be very difficult indeed. Nonetheless, you may find this list of salicylate-containing foods useful.

Children with Autistic Spectrum Disorders (ASD) have a number of metabolic imbalances, and one in particular relates to an inability to handle salicylates properly. The process within the body called sulphation may be impaired due to a lack of an enzyme called Phenol-Sulpho-Transferase-P (PST). PST links a sulfur molecule to a variety of substances, including salicylate, making them water soluble so that they can be detoxified. If this does not happen, then substances like salicylates can build up and become toxic in the body.

Food colorings seem to inhibit PST, thus increasing the risk of inducing toxicity in individuals because they become unable to detoxify certain chemicals in their diet.

There may also be problems with sulfation processes themselves, which would require making sure you get adequate molybdenum in your diet.

Salicylates are found in the following: natural flavorings and colorings, aspirin and products containing aspirin and salicylic acid.

High Salicylate Foods

Fruits

Avocado

Apples (most varieties)

Apricots

Berries (all)

Cherries

Dates

Grapes (also raisins, currants, sultanas)

Grapefruit

Guava

Kiwi

Melon (water and Cantaloupe)

Nectarines

Oranges

Peaches

Pineapple

Plums

Prunes

Tangerines

Vegetables

Alfalfa sprouts

Chicory

Cucumbers and cucumber pickles

Endive

Gherkins

Peppers (bell and chili)

Radish

Tomatoes and tomato products

Watercress

Zucchini

Seeds, Nuts

Almonds

Brazil nuts

Macadamia nuts

Peanuts with skins on

Pine nuts

Pistachio

Sesame seeds

Herbs, Spices, Condiments

Bayleaf

Cardamom, caraway, cayenne, cumin, curry

Cinnamon, nutmeg

Chili powder, garam masala, turmeric

Cider and cider vinegar (apples)

Cloves

Dill, mint, oregano, rosemary, sage, tarragon, thyme and mixed herbs

Five spice

Ginger

Marmite

Mustard

Paprika

Pepper (black and white)

Beverages

Coffee

Peppermint tea

Port, rum

Tea (all brands)

Wine and wine vinegar (grapes)

Other

Molasses and honey

Rose hips and acerola (often found in vitamins)

Wintergreen ointment (methyl salicylate)

Foods indicated in **BOLD** are found in practice to be the most problematic where salicylate sensitivity exists. Avoid all these foods for 4–6 weeks, and as many of the remaining ones as possible (particularly grapefruit, kiwi, and pineapple).

Foods indicated in *ITALICS* below represent 'safe' foods (they contain negligible or low levels of salicylates). The other foods listed contain moderate amounts of salicylates – eat sparingly.

Fruits

Apple – *green golden delicious, peeled*

Apple – red golden delicious, peeled

Banana

Fresh figs

Lemon

Lime

Mango

Passion fruit

Pear – peeled

Paw paw

Pomegranate

Rhubarb

Tamarillo

Vegetables

Asparagus

Bamboo shoots

Beans and peas

Beetroot

Broccoli

Brown lentils

Brussels sprouts

Cabbage

Carrot

Cauliflower

Celery

Chive

Leek

Lettuce

Mushroom

Onion

Parsnip

Potato (peeled)

Red cabbage

Spinach

Squash

Sweet potato

Seeds, Nuts

Cashews

Coconut

Hazel nuts

Poppy seed

Walnuts

Herbs, Spices, Condiments

Garlic

Malt vinegar

Parsley

Saffron

Soy sauce

Vanilla

Beverages

Camomile tea

Dandelion coffee

Decaffeinated coffee

Pear juice

Gin, whisky, vodka

Other

Carob

Cold pressed oils such as sunflower

Supplementation to support sulfation (which would include the trace mineral molybdenum) also improves your salicylate tolerance. This is something that would be considered if you see improvements after eliminating salicylate-rich foods.

Sources

Feingold program: http://www.feingold.org.dietshell

The list above is based on research by Anne Swain. Anne is head dietician at the Allergy Unit in the Department of Clinical Immunology at Sydney's Royal Prince Alfred Hospital. She is a key member of the team that leads the world in assessing and managing food intolerances. She is co-author of *Friendly Food, The Simplified Elimination Diet* and *Salicylates, Amines and Glutamates.*

The Feingold website refers to Anne's research as 'definitive'. Her research is based on salicylate levels per 100g of food, which would suggest that the herbs and spice list on page 317 may not be such a problem (who eats 100g of mustard or oregano?).

The foods in **bold** on pages 316–17 represent those found by the Feingold program to be the most problematic. There are three additional foods that I would empha-size on this list – grapefruit, kiwi, and pineapple. These contain high amounts of salicylates according to Anne Swain's research, although they are not flagged up on the Feingold program.

Lastly, while bananas are very low in salicylates, they contain high levels of phenolics so they should be consumed sparingly. Cocoa is another food that is low in salicylates but high in phenolics, so it has been left off the list completely.

Those with autism or ADHD have been shown to have low levels of the enzyme PST (phenol sulfo transferase) needed to metabolize high-phenolic substances. Salicylates depress PST levels even further. Hence, as well as trying a diet without high-salicylate foods (in order to raise PST levels), avoiding high phenolic foods such as bananas is also judicious (as this will take stress off your enzyme system).

References

Introduction

American Academy of Allergy, Asthma and Immunology (AAAAI), *The Allergy Report: Science-based Findings on the Diagnosis and Treatment of Allergic Disorders* (1996–2001)

The International Study of Asthma and Allergies in Childhood (ISAAC) Steering Committee, 'Worldwide variation in prevalence of symptoms of asthma, allergic rhinoconjunctivitis, and atopic eczema: ISAAC', *Lancet* 1998; 351: 1225–32

Chapter One

Bryan, W. T. K. and Bryan, M. P. 'Clinical examples of resolution of some idiopathic and other chronic disease by careful allergic management', *Layrngoscope* 1972; 82: 1231–38

Murray, M. *The Healing Power of Foods* (Prima Publishing, 1993)

Chapter Two

Abrahams, N., PhD, Berni-Klerck, L., Sharma, R., Gaier, H. *The use of a Cellular Mediator Release Assay (FACT) for the Identification of Food Sensitivity in Clinical Practice*

Barrie, S. 'Food Allergies', *Natural Medicine Journal* August/September 1998: 6–17

Buckley, R. 'Food Allergy', *Journal of American Medical Association* 1982; 248: 2627–29

Hamburger, R. *Proceedings of First International Symposium on Food Allergy,* Vancouver BC, 1982

Herman, P. M. and Drost, L. M. 'Evaluating the clinical relevance of food sensitivity tests: a single-subject experiment', *Alternative Medicine Review* 2004; 9(2): 198–207

Jones, V. A. et al. 'Food intolerance: a major factor in the pathogenesis of irritable bowel syndrome', *Lancet* 1982; 2: 1115–17

Perelmutter, L. 'Non-IgE mediated atopic disease', *Annals of Allergy* 1984; 52: 64–69

Chapter Three

Andre, F., Andre, C., Colin, L., Cacaraci, F., Cavagna, S. 'Role of new allergens and of allergens consumed in the increased incidence of food sensitizations in France', *Toxicology* 1994 Sep 22; 93(1): 77–83

Ansaldi-Balocco, N., Santini, B., Sarchi, C. 'Efficacy of pancreatic enzyme supplementation in children with cystic fibrosis: comparison of two preparations by random crossover study and a retrospective study of the same patients at two different ages', *J Pediatr Gastroenterol Nutr* 1988; 7 Suppl 1: S40–5

Anthony, H., Collins, C. E., Davidson, G., Mews, C., Robinson, P., Shepherd, R., Stapleton, D. 'Pancreatic enzyme replacement therapy in cystic fibrosis: Australian guidelines', *J Paediatr Child Health* Apr 1999; 35(2): 125–9

Braga, M., Cristallo, M., De Franchis, R., Mangiagalli, A., Agape, D., Primignani, M., Di Carlo, V. 'Correction of malnutrition and maldigestion with enzyme supplementation in patients with surgical suppression of exocrine pancreatic function', *Surg Gynecol Obstet* Dec 1988; 167(6): 485–92

Bray G. 'Hypochlorhydria and childhood asthma', *Quart J Medicine* 1941; 27: 113

Brostoff, J. and Gamlin, L. *The Complete Guide to Food Allergy and Intolerance* (Bloomsbury Publishing Ltd, 1990)

Brudnak, M. *The Probiotic Solution* (Dragon Door Publications, 2003)

Bueno, H. *Uninvited Guests* (Keats, 1996)

Delhaye, M., Meuris, S., Gohimont, A. C., Buedts, K., Cremer, M. 'Comparative evaluation of a high lipase pancreatic enzyme preparation and a standard pancreatic supplement for treating exocrine pancreatic insufficiency in chronic pancreatitis', *Eur J Gastroenterol Hepatol* Jul 1996; 8(7): 699–703

Desser, L., Holomanova, D., Zavadova, E., Pavelka, K., Mohr, T., Herbacek, I. 'Oral therapy with proteolytic enzymes decreases excessive TGF-beta levels in human blood', *Cancer Chemother Pharmacol* Jul 2001; 47 Suppl: S10–5

Dominguez-Munoz, J. E., Birckelbach, U., Glasbrenner, B., Sauerbruch, T., Malfertheiner, P. 'Effect of oral pancreatic enzyme administration on digestive function in healthy subjects: comparison between two enzyme preparations', *Aliment Pharmacol Ther* Apr 1997; 11(2): 403–8

Ducluzeau, R. and Bensaada, M. 'Comparative effect of a single or continuous administration of *Saccharomyces boulardii* on the establishment of various strains of candida in the digestive tract of gnotobiotic mice', *Ann Microbiol* 1982; 133: 491–501

Eastham, E. J., Douglas, A. P., Watson, A. J. 'Diagnosis of *Giardi lamblia* infection as a cause of diarrhoea', *Lancet* 1976: 950–1

Hamilton, J. R. 'Retinal abnormalities with chronic pancreatitis', *New England Journal of Medicine* 1981; 302: 1316

Hemmings, W. A., Williams, E. W. 'Transport of large breakdown products of dietary protein through the gut wall', *Gut* 1978; 19: 715

Howden, C. W., Hunt, R. M. *Gut* 1987; 28: 96

Hussain Quadri, S. M., Al-Okaili, G. A., Al-Dayel, F. 'Clinical significance of Blastocystis hominis', *J. Clin Microbiol* 1989; 27 (11): 2407–9

Galland, L., Lee, M., Bueno, H., Heimowitz, C. '*Giardia lamblia* infection as a cause of chronic fatigue', *J. Nutr. Med* 1(1), 190: 27–32

Gittelman, L. Guess *What Came to Dinner?* (Avery Publishing, 1993)

Greenberger, N. J. 'Enzymatic therapy in patients with chronic pancreatitis', *Gastroenterol Clin North Am* Sep 1999; 28(3): 687–93

Kain, K. C., Noble, M. A., Freeman, H. J., Barteluk, R. 'Epidemiology and clinical features associated with Blastocystis hominis infection', *Diagn. Microbiol. Infect. Dis* 1987; 8(4): 234–44

Kreuning, J., Bosman, F., Kuiper, G. et al. *J Clin Pathol* 1978; 31: 69

Layer, P., Keller, J., Lankisch, P. G. 'Pancreatic enzyme replacement therapy', *Curr Gastroenterol Rep* Apr 2001; 3(2): 101–8

Layer, P. and Keller, J. 'Lipase supplementation therapy: standards, alternatives, and perspectives', *Pancreas* Jan 2003; 26(1): 1–7

Lipski, E. *Digestive Wellness* (Keats, 1996)

Madden, J. A. J., Hunter, J. O. *Brit J. Nutr* 2002; 88(1): S67

McFarland, L. V., Elmer, G. W. 'Biotherapeutic agents: past, present and future', *Microecology Ther* 1995; 23: 46–73

Modlin, I. M. Goldenring, J. R. Lawton, G. P. and Hunt, R. *Am. J. Gastroenterol* 1994; 89(3): 308

Newey, H., Smyth, D. H. 1959. 'Intestinal absorption of dipeptides', *J. Physiol* 1959; 145: 48

Plummer, N. 'The Unseen Epidemic: The Linked Syndromes of Achlohydria and Atrophic Gastritis', *Townsend Letter for Doctors and Patients*, July 2004: 89–94

Rigothier, M. C., Maccario, J. and Gayral, P. 'Inhibitory activity of saccharomyces yeasts on the adhesion of Entameoba histolytica trophozoites to human erythrocytes in vitro', *Parasitol Res* 1994; 80: 10–15

Russo, A. R., Stone, S. L., Taplin, M. E., Snapper, H. J., Doern, G. V. 'Presumptive evidence for Blastocystis hominis as a cause of colitis', *Arch. Intern. Med* 1988; 148(5): 1064

Villako, K., Tamm, A., Savisaar, E., Ruttas, M. *Scand J Gastoenterol* 1987; 11: 817

Walker, W. A. 'Uptake and transport of macromolecules by the intestine – possible role in clinical disorders', *Gastroenterol* 1974; 67: 531

Zierdt, C. *Clin. Microbiol. Rev* Jan 1991; vol 4: 61–79

Chapter Four

Jones, V. A. et al. 'Food intolerance: a major factor in the pathogenesis of irritable bowel syndrome', *Lancet* 1982; 2: 1115–17

Chapter Five

Andre, C., Andre, F., Colin, L., Cavagna, S. 'Measurement of intestinal permeability to mannitol and lactulose as a means of diagnosing food allergy and evaluating therapeutic effectiveness of disodium cromoglycate', *Ann Allergy* 1987; 59: 127–30

Benard, A., Desreumeaux, P., Huglo, D., et al. 'Increased intestinal permeability in bronchial asthma', *J Allergy Clin Immunol* 1996; 97: 1173–78

Berg, R. D. 'Bacterial translocation from the gastrointestinal tract', *J. Med* 1992; 23: 217–44

Bjarnson, I. 'Intestinal permeability', *Gut* 1994; 35: S18–S22

Bjarnson, I., Peters, T. J. 'Influence of anti-rheumatic drugs on gut permeability and on the gut associated lymphoid tissue', *Baillieres Clin Rheumatol* 1996; 10: 165–76

Bjarnson, I., Williams, P., Smethurst, P. et al. 'Effect of non-steroidal anti-inflammatory drugs and prostaglandins on the permeability of the human small intestine', *Gut* 1986; 27: 1292–97

Bjarnson, I., Williams, P., So, A. et al. 'Intestinal permeability and inflammation in rheumatoid arthritis: effects of non-steroidal anti-inflammatory drugs', *Lancet* 1984; 2(8413): 1171–74

Bjarnson, I., Zanelli, G., Smith, T. et al. 'The pathogenesis and consequences of non-steroidal anti-inflammatory drug-induced small intestinal inflammation in man', *Scan J Rheumatology* 1987; 64: S55–S62

Bridges, S. R., Anderson, J. W., Deakins, D. A. et al. 'Oat bran increases serum acetate of hypercholesterolemic men', *Am J Clin Nutr* 1992; 56: 455–59

Catanzarro, J. A., Green, L. 'Microbial ecology and probiotics in human medicine (Part II)', *Alt Med Rev* 1997; 2: 296–305

Cobden, I., Rothwell, J., Axon, A. T. R. 'Intestinal permeability and screening tests for celiac disease', *Gut* 1980; 21: 512–18

Crowe, S. E., Perdue, M. H. 'Functional abnormalities in the intestine associated with mucosal mast cell activation', *Reg Immunol* 1992; 4: 113–17

Hangee-Bauer, C. 'Lactobacilli and human health' in *A Textbook of Natural Medicine* (Seattle, WA: Bastyr University Publications, 1985): V: Latob-1–5

Katz, K. D., Hollander, R., Vadheim, C. M. et al. 'Intestinal permeability in patients with Crohn's disease and their healthy relatives', *Gastroenterology* 1989; 97: 927–31

Keller, S. D. E., Weiss, J. M., Schleifer, S. J. et al. 'Suppression of immunity by stress: Effect of graded series of stressors on lymphocyte stimulation in the rat', *Science* 1981; 213: 1397–1400; Ader, R. (ed), *Psychoimmunology* (New York: Academic Press, 1981)

Kennedy, M. J., Volz, P. A. 'Ecology of Candida albicans gut colonization: Inhibition of Candida adhesion, colonization and dissemination from the gastrointestinal tract by bacterial antagonism', *Infect Immun* 1985; 49: 654–63

Lichtenberger, L. M., Wang, Z., Romero, J. J. et al. 'Non-steroidal anti-inflammatory drugs (NSAIDs) associate with zwitterionic phospholipids: Insight into the mechanism and reversal of NSAID-induced gastrointestinal injury', *Nat Med* 1995; 1: 154–58

Mack, D. R., Flick, J. A., Durie, P. R. et al. 'Correlation of intestinal permeability with exocrine pancreatic dysfunction', *J. Pediatr* 1992; 120: 696–701

Maln, M., Suomalainen, H., Saxelin, M., Isolauri, E. 'Promotion of IgA immune response in patients with Crohn's disease by oral bacteriotherapy with *Lactobacillus* GG', *Ann Nutr Metab* 1996; 40: 137–45

Martinez-Gonzalez, O., Cantero-Hinjosa, J., Paule-Sastre, P. et al. 'Intestinal permeability in patients with ankylosing spondylitis and their healthy relatives', Br. *J. Rheumatol* 1994; 33: 644–47

May, T., Mackie, R. I., Fahey, G. C, Jr et al. 'Effect of fiber source on short-chain fatty acid production and on the growth and toxin production of *Clostridium difficile*', *Scand J Gastroenterol* 1994; 29: 916–22

Miller, A. L. 'The pathogenesis, clinical implications, and treatment of intestinal hyperpermeability', *Alt Med Rev* 1997; 2: 330–45

Moneret-Vautrin, D. A., Kanny, G., Thevenin, F. 'Asthma caused by food allergy', *Rev Med. Interne* 196; 17: 551–57

Murphy, M. S., Eastham, E. J., Nelson, R. et al. 'Intestinal permeability in Crohn's disease', *Arch Dis Child* 1989; 64: 321–25

Olaison, G., Sjodahl, R., Tagesson, C. 'Abnormal intestinal permeability in Crohn's Disease', *Scan J Gastroenterol* 1990; 25: 321–28

Paganelli, R., Fagiolo, U., Cancian, M., Scala, E. 'Intestinal permeability in patients with chronic urticaria-angioedema with and without arthralgia', *Ann Allergy* 1991; 66: 181–84

Pearce, F. L., Befus, A. D., Bienenstock, J. 'Mucosal mast cells. III. Effect of quercetin and other flavonoids on antigen-induced histamine secretion from rat intestinal mast cells', *J Allergy Clin Immunol* 1984; 73: 819–23

Peeters, M., Geypens, B., Claus, D. et al. 'Clustering of increased small intestinal permeability in families with Crohn's disease', *Gastroenterology* 1997; 113: 802–7

Saadia, R. and Lipman, J. 'Antibiotics and the gut', *Eur J Surg* 1996; 576: S39–S41

Smith, M. D., Gibson, R. A., Brooks, P. M. 'Abnormal bowel permeability in ankylosing spondylitis and rheumatoid arthritis', *J. Rheumatol* 1985; 12: 299–305

Tatsuno, K. 'Intestinal permeability in children with food allergy', *Arerugi* 1989; 38: 1311–18

Taylor, B., Norman, A. P., Orgel, C. R. et al. 'Transient IgA deficiency and pathogenesis of infantile atopy', *Lancet* 1973; ii: 111–13

Teahon, K., Smethurst, P., Levi, A. J. et al. 'Intestinal permeability in patients with Crohn's disease and their first degree relatives', *Gut* 1992; 33: 320–23

Walker, W. A. 'Uptake and transport of macromolecules by the intestine – possible role in clinical disorders', *Gastroenterology* 1974; 67: 531–50

Ward, P. B., Young, G. P. 'Dynamics of *Clostridum difficile* infection. Control using diet', *Adv Exp Med Biol* 1997; 412: 63–75

Wyatt, J., Vogelsgang, H., Hubl, W. et al. 'Intestinal permeability and the prediction of relapse in Crohn's disease', *Lancet* 1993; 341: 1437–39

Chapter Six

Abrahams, N. PhD, Berni-Klerck, L., Sharma, R., Gaier, H. *The use of a Cellular Mediator Release Assay (FACT) for the Identification of Food Sensitivity in Clinical Practice*

Blair, D. M., Hangee-Bauer, C. S., Calabrese, C. 'Intestinal candidiasis, *L. acidophilus supplementation* and Crook's questionnaire', *J Naturopathic Med* 1991; 2: 33–37

Braly, J. and Torbet, L. *Dr Braly's Food Allergy & Nutrition Revolution* (Keats, 1992)

Crook, W. G. *The Yeast Connection: A Medical Breakthrough* (Jackson, TN: Professional Books, 1984)

Katsuki, A., Sumida, Y. et al. 'Serum levels of TNFa are increased in obese patients with non-insulin-dependant diabetes mellitus', *J Clin Endocrinol Metab* 1998; 83(3): 859–62

Bibliography

American Academy of Allergy, Asthma and Immunology (AAAAI). *The Allergy Report: Science-based Findings on the Diagnosis and Treatment of Allergic Disorders* (1996–2001)

Atkinson W. Sheldon T. A., Shaath N. & Whorwhell P. J., 'Food elimination based on IgG antibodies in irritable bowel syndrome: a randomised controlled trial', *Gut*, 2004; 53: 1459–64

Brostoff, Dr J. and Gamlin, L. *The Complete Guide to Food Allergy and Intolerance* (Bloomsbury, 1990)

Buist, R. *Food Intolerance – What It Is and How to Cope with It* (Prism Press, 1984)

Clarke, T. W. 'The relation of allergy to chocolate problems in children: a survey', *Psychiatric Quarterly* 24 (1950): 21

Coca, Arthur F. *The Pulse Test: Easy Allergy Detection* (NY: Arco Publishing, 1956)

——. The Pulse Test (NY: ARC Books, 1959): 17

Crook, W. G. *Your Child and Allergy* (Jackson, TN: Professional Books, 1973): 20

——. *Can Your Child Read? Is He Hyperactive?* (Jackson, TN: Professional Books, 1977)

Davison, H. M. 'Cerebral allergy', *Southern Med. Journal* 42 (1949): 712

Duke, W. W. 'Food allergy as a cause of abdominal pain', *Arch Intern Med* 28 (1921): 151

——. 'Ménière's syndrome caused by allergies', *Journal of the American Medical Association* 81 (1923): 2179

Feingold, Ben F. *Introduction to Clinical Allergy* (Springfield, IL: Charles C. Thomas, 1972)

Hoobler, B. R. 'Some early symptoms suggesting protein sensitization in infancy', *Am Journal of Diseases Children* 12 (1916): 129

The International Study of Asthma and Allergies in Childhood (ISAAC) Steering Committee. 'Worldwide variation in prevalence of symptoms of asthma, allergic rhinoconjunctivitis, and atopic eczema: ISAAC', *Lancet* (1998) 351: 1225–32

King, D. S. and Mandell, M. A. 'Double-blind study of allergic cerebral-viscero-somatic malfunctions evoked by provocative sublingual challenges with allergic extracts: statistical confirmation of the induction of psychological (mental) and somatic symptoms by provocative testing', *Proceedings of the 12th Advanced Seminar in Clinical Ecology*, Key Biscayne, Florida, October, 1978. *See also*: King, D. S. 'Effects of sublingual testing: a double-blind study', *Proceedings of the 13th Advanced Seminar in Clinical Ecology*, San Diego, October, 1979

Kittler, F. J. and Baldwin, D. G. 'The role of allergic factors in the child with minimal brain dysfunction', *Annals of Allergy* 23 (1970): 203

Lowell, Jax Peters. *Against the Grain* (NY: Henry Holt & Company Inc., 1995)

MacKarness, Richard. *Eating Dangerously: The Hazards of Hidden Allergies* (NY: Harcourt, Brace Jovanovich, 1979)

Miller, J. B. 'A double-blind study of food extract injection therapy: a preliminary report', *Annals of Allergy* 38 (1977): 185

Moyer, K. E. 'The physiology of violence: allergy and aggression', *Psychology Today* July 1975: 76–79

O'Shea, J. 'Sublingual immunotherapy of hyperactive children with food, chemical inhalant allergens: a double-blind study', *Proceedings of the 12th Advanced Seminar in Clinical Ecology*, Key Biscayne, Florida, October, 1978

Pert, Candace, *The Molecules of Emotion* (NY: Scribner, 1997)

Pfeiffer, C., PhD, MD. *Nutrition and Mental Illness* (Healing Arts Press, 1987)

Philpott, W. H. *Ecologic Medicine Manual* (mimeographed) (Oklahoma City, 1975): 2–3

Philpott, W. H., MD and Kalita, D. K., PhD, *Brain Allergies* (2nd edn; Keats Publishing, 2000)

Randolph, Theron G. *Human Ecology and Susceptibility to the Chemical Environment* (Springfield, IL: Charles C. Thomas, 1962)

——. 'Fatigue and weakness of allergic origin (Allergic Toxemia) to be differentiated from nervous fatigue and neurasthenia', *Annals of Allergy* 3 (1945): 418

Rapaport, H. G. and Flint, S. H. 'Is there a relationship between allergy and learning disabilities?', *J. School Health* 46 (1976)

Rapp, Doris J. 'Does diet affect hyperactivity?', *J. Learning Disability* 11 (1978): 383

Rinkel, H. J. 'Food allergy: the role of food allergy in internal medicine', *Annals of Allergy* 2 (1944): 115

Rinkel, H. J., Randolph, T. G. and Zeller, M. *Food Allergy* (Springfield, IL: Charles C. Thomas, 1951)

Roth, June. *The Food/Depression Connection: Dietary Control of Allergy-Based Mood Swings* (Chicago: Contemporary Books, 1978)

Rowe, A. H. *Food Allergy* (Philadelphia: Lea & Febiger, 1931)

——. *Elimination Diets and the Patient's Allergies* (Henry Kimpton, 1944)

——. 'Allergic toxicemia and fatigue', *Annals of Allergy* 8 (1950): 72

Rowe, A. H. and Rowe, A. H. Jr. *Food Allergy* (Springfield, IL: Charles C. Thomas, 1972)

Schauss, A. *Diet, Crime and Delinquency* (rev. edn; Parker House, 1981)

Selye, H. *The Stress of Life* (McGraw-Hill Education, 1978)

Speer, F. 'Allergic tension-fatigue in children', *Annals of Allergy* 12 (1954): 168

Swanson, J. 'Behavioural responses to artificial colour', presented at the 2nd International Food Allergy Symposium, the American College of Allergists, Mexico City, Mexico, 1978

William, J. J., Cram, D. M., Tausig, F. T. and Webster, E. 'Relative effects of drugs and diet on hyperactive behaviours: an experimental study', *Pediatrics* 61 (1978): 811

Winkleman, N. W. and Moore, M. T. 'Allergy and nervous diseases', *J. Nervous and Mental Diseases* 93 (1941): 736

Resources

Whole Foods Market® have stores all over the country for organic and allergy-free foods. Availability will depend on your local store. The website advertises many gluten- and dairy-free products including cereals, flours, grains, seeds, baked goods and mixes; ingredients such as egg replacer, cornstarch, baking powder, bouillon and breadcrumbs; staple foods such as pasta, dairy-free beverages and products and, for the occasional luxury, a selection of chocolate.

Whole Foods Market, Inc.
550 Bowie Street
Austin, TX 78703-4644
Tel: 512-477-4455
Fax: 512-482-7000
website: www.wholefoodsmarket.com

Useful information and help can be obtained from the following organization:

Institute for Functional Medicine (IFM)

4411 Pt. Fosdick Drive NW

Suite 305

PO Box 1697

Gig Harbor

Washington State 98335

Tel: 800-228-0622

Fax: 253-853-6766

email: client_services@fxmed.com

website: www.functionalmedicine.org

The Purpose Statement of the IFM is:

> *The Institute provides continuing medical education for physicians and other healthcare professionals, publishes books and other educational materials, and offers clinicians a Forum for the shared exploration of emerging research and clinical applications to improve patient care and outcomes.*

If you wish to seek the help of a practitioner, I strongly recommend that you visit someone trained in Functional Medicine who will take a holistic view of you and your health. To find a Functional Medicine Practitioner, visit:

http://www.functionalmedicine.org/findfmphysician/index.asp

Index